Evaluating Hearing Loss for Individuals with Cochlear Implants

Committee on Evaluating Hearing Loss for
Individuals with Cochlear Implants

Board on Health Care Services

Health and Medicine Division

A Consensus Study Report of

The National Academies of
SCIENCES • ENGINEERING • MEDICINE

THE NATIONAL ACADEMIES PRESS
Washington, DC
www.nap.edu

THE NATIONAL ACADEMIES PRESS   500 Fifth Street, NW   Washington, DC 20001

This activity was supported by a contract between the National Academy of Sciences and the U.S. Social Security Administration (Contract No. 28321318D00060015). Any opinions, findings, conclusions, or recommendations expressed in this publication do not necessarily reflect the views of any organization or agency that provided support for the project.

International Standard Book Number-13: 978-0-309-26454-9
International Standard Book Number-10: 0-309-26454-5
Digital Object Identifier: https://doi.org/10.17226/26057

Additional copies of this publication are available from the National Academies Press, 500 Fifth Street, NW, Keck 360, Washington, DC 20001; (800) 624-6242 or (202) 334-3313; http://www.nap.edu.

Copyright 2021 by the National Academy of Sciences. All rights reserved.

Printed in the United States of America

Suggested citation: National Academies of Sciences, Engineering, and Medicine. 2021. *Evaluating hearing loss for individuals with cochlear implants*. Washington, DC: The National Academies Press. https://doi.org/10.17226/26057.

The National Academies of
SCIENCES • ENGINEERING • MEDICINE

The National Academy of Sciences was established in 1863 by an Act of Congress, signed by President Lincoln, as a private nongovernment institution to advise the nation on issues related to science and technology. Members are elected by their peers for outstanding contributions to research. Dr. Marcia McNutt is president.

The National Academy of Engineering was established in 1964 under the charter of the National Academy of Sciences to bring the practices of engineering to advising the nation. Members are elected by their peers for extraordinary contributions to engineering. Dr. John L. Anderson is president.

The National Academy of Medicine (formerly the Institute of Medicine) was established in 1970 under the charter of the National Academy of Sciences to advise the nation on medical and health issues. Members are elected by their peers for distinguished contributions to medicine and health. Dr. Victor J. Dzau is president.

The three Academies work together as the **National Academies of Sciences, Engineering, and Medicine** to provide independent, objective analysis and advice to the nation and conduct other activities to solve complex problems and inform public-policy decisions. The National Academies also encourage education and research, recognize outstanding contributions to knowledge, and increase public understanding in matters of science, engineering, and medicine.

Learn more about the National Academies of Sciences, Engineering, and Medicine at **www.nationalacademies.org**.

The National Academies of
SCIENCES · ENGINEERING · MEDICINE

Consensus Study Reports published by the National Academies of Sciences, Engineering, and Medicine document the evidence-based consensus on studies' statements of task by committees of experts. Reports typically include findings, conclusions, and recommendations based on information gathered by the committees and the committees' deliberations. Each report has been subjected to a rigorous and independent peer-review process and represents the position of the National Academies on its statement of task.

Proceedings published by the National Academies of Sciences, Engineering, and Medicine chronicle the presentations and discussions at workshops, symposia, or other events convened by the National Academies. The statements and opinions contained in proceedings are those of the participants and are not endorsed by other participants, the planning committee, or the National Academies.

For information about other products and activities of the National Academies, please visit www.nationalacademies.org/about/whatwedo.

COMMITTEE ON EVALUATING HEARING LOSS FOR INDIVIDUALS WITH COCHLEAR IMPLANTS

JUDITH GREEN-McKENZIE (*Chair*), Professor and Chief, Division of Occupational and Environmental Medicine, University of Pennsylvania Perelman School of Medicine
RENÉ H. GIFFORD, Professor of Hearing and Speech Sciences and Director of the Cochlear Implant Program, Vanderbilt University Medical Center
FRANK R. LIN, Professor of Otolaryngology and Director of the Cochlear Center for Hearing and Public Health, Johns Hopkins University
KNASHAWN H. MORALES, Associate Professor, Department of Biostatistics, Epidemiology and Informatics, University of Pennsylvania Perelman School of Medicine
SARAH F. POISSANT, Associate Professor and Acting Chair, Communication Disorders Department, University of Massachusetts Amherst
NICHOLAS S. REED, Audiologist and Assistant Professor of Epidemiology, Johns Hopkins Bloomberg School of Public Health
GRETA C. STAMPER, Audiology Division Chair and Assistant Professor of Audiology, Mayo Clinic Florida
TERESA A. ZWOLAN, Professor of Otolaryngology and Director of the Cochlear Implant Program, University of Michigan

Consultant

KARL R. WHITE, Professor of Psychology and Director of the National Center for Hearing Assessment and Management, Utah State University

Study Staff

CAROLYN FULCO, Scholar
BERNICE CHU, Program Officer
BLAKE REICHMUTH, Associate Program Officer
JOSEPH GOODMAN, Senior Program Assistant
SHARYL NASS, Senior Director, Board on Health Care Services

Reviewers

This Consensus Study Report was reviewed in draft form by individuals chosen for their diverse perspectives and technical expertise. The purpose of this independent review is to provide candid and critical comments that will assist the National Academies of Sciences, Engineering, and Medicine in making each published report as sound as possible and to ensure that it meets the institutional standards for quality, objectivity, evidence, and responsiveness to the study charge. The review comments and draft manuscript remain confidential to protect the integrity of the deliberative process.

We thank the following individuals for their review of this report:

JULIE G. ARENBERG, Harvard Medical School
BRUCE J. GANTZ, University of Iowa
HOWARD H. GOLDMAN, University of Maryland School
    of Medicine
SANDRA GORDON-SALANT, University of Maryland
MICHAEL MERZENICH, University of California, San Francisco
STEPHANIE J. SJOBLAD, University of North Carolina at
    Chapel Hill

Although the reviewers listed above provided many constructive comments and suggestions, they were not asked to endorse the conclusions or recommendations of this report nor did they see the final draft before its release. The review of this report was overseen by **DAN G. BLAZER,**

Duke University Medical Center, and **BRUCE N. CALONGE,** University of Colorado School of Medicine. They were responsible for making certain that an independent examination of this report was carried out in accordance with the standards of the National Academies and that all review comments were carefully considered. Responsibility for the final content rests entirely with the authoring committee and the National Academies.

Contents

ACRONYMS AND ABBREVIATIONS — xi

SUMMARY — 1

1 INTRODUCTION — 15
   Statement of Task, 17
   Approach to the Task, 19
   Cochlear Implants, 19
   Introduction to the Hearing in Noise Test, 23
   Organization of the Report, 24
   References, 25

2 CONSIDERATIONS FOR EVALUATING
   HEARING FUNCTION — 29
   Auditory Processing: Detection and Perception, 29
   Hearing Test Characteristics, 31
   Presentation Level and Test Setup, 32
   Introduction to Speech Tests, 39
   References, 44

3 CHARACTERISTICS AND LIMITATIONS OF THE
   HEARING IN NOISE TEST — 49
   Background, 49
   Development of the Hearing in Noise Test, 50

Administration of the Hearing in Noise Test, 52
Salient Characteristics of the Hearing in Noise Test, 52
The Hearing in Noise Test as a Test for Individuals with
    Cochlear Implants, 54
Limitations of the Hearing in Noise Test, 55
References, 56

4 CHARACTERISTICS OF HEARING AND SPEECH TESTS   59
Cross-Cutting Issues, 61
Sentence Tests, 62
Word Tests, 69
Considerations Beyond Auditory Testing, 74
Conclusions and Recommendation, 78
References, 79

**5 EVALUATING HEARING ABILITY IN PERSONS
    WITH COCHLEAR IMPLANTS WITH SINGLE-SIDED
    DEAFNESS OR ASYMMETRIC HEARING LOSS   85**
Introduction, 86
Special Consideration in the Testing and Treatment of Persons
    with Bilateral But Unequal Hearing Loss, 88
Correlation Between Hearing Loss in the Less-Affected Ear and
    Recovery Time or Treatment in the More-Affected Ear, 91
Single-Sided Deafness, Asymmetric Hearing Loss, and Social
    Security Disability, 93
Testing Hearing Ability in Persons with Single-Sided Deafness
    or Asymmetric Hearing Loss Receiving a Cochlear Implant, 94
Proxies for the Hearing in Noise Test for Individuals with
    Single-Sided Deafness or Asymmetric Hearing Loss, 95
References, 95

6 TEST COMPARISONS AND RECOMMENDATIONS   99
Test Comparisons, 100
Alternative Measures for the Hearing in Noise Test
    Equivalence, 102
Summary and Recommendations, 103
References, 107

Acronyms and Abbreviations

0° azimuth	angle in relation to the listener that is directly in front of the listener
AHL	asymmetric hearing loss
AzBio	Arizona Biomedical Sentences Test
BKB	Bamford, Kowal, and Bench
BKB-SIN	Bamford-Kowal-Bench Speech-in-Noise Test
CID	Central Institute for the Deaf
CNC	consonant–nucleus–consonant (refers to the Maryland CNC word test)
CPT	current procedural terminology
CROS	contralateral routing of signal
CUNY	City University of New York
dB	decibel (a unit of measure for sound level)
dB A	decibels with A-weighted sound levels (designed to mimic the spectral range and audibility curves, in dB SPL, of human hearing)
dB HL	decibel hearing level (the decibel measure displayed on an audiometer, normalized so that 0 dB HL = average normal for all frequencies)

dB SPL	decibel sound pressure level (the decibel measure that most people are familiar with and referencing the pressure of the measured displacement of air molecules relative to the surrounding or ambient air pressure)
DI	disability insurance
EPA	U.S. Environmental Protection Agency
EXT A or B	external or auxiliary input setting for an audiometer
FDA	U.S. Food and Drug Administration
HINT	Hearing in Noise Test
HINT-C	Hearing in Noise Test-Children
Hz	Hertz (a measure of frequency [pitch], describing number of cycles per second)
IA	interaural attenuation
IEEE	Institute of Electrical and Electronics Engineers
LNT	Lexical Neighborhood Test
MLNT	Multisyllabic Neighborhood Test
MLV	monitored live voice
MSTB	Minimum Speech Test Battery
NCT	National Clinical Trial
NU-6	Northwestern University Test Number 6
OR	odds ratio
PBK	Phonetically Balanced Kindergarten (a word test)
PTA	pure tone average
QuickSIN	Quick Speech in Noise Test
S/B	signal-to-babble ratio
SIN	Speech in Noise Test
SLM	sound level meter
SNR	signal-to-noise ratio
SPL	sound pressure level
SRM	spatial release from masking
SRT	speech recognition threshold

SSA	U.S. Social Security Administration
SSD	single-sided deafness
SSDI	Social Security Disability Insurance
SSI	Supplemental Security Income
T Level	threshold level
UHL	unilateral hearing loss
VU meter	volume unit meter (a device that displays a representation of the signal level)
WIN	Words in Noise Test

Summary

The U.S. Social Security Administration (SSA) administers the Social Security Disability Insurance (SSDI) program and the Supplemental Security Income (SSI) program. Those programs provide disability benefits to individuals who qualify due to a disability. Once SSA establishes the presence of a severe medically determinable impairment, it determines whether the impairment meets or equals the criteria in the *Listing of Impairments* (the Listings), which are lists of medical conditions that qualify a candidate for disability benefits regardless of the applicant's age, education, or work experience. If an individual does not meet Listings-level criteria, they can still qualify for disability further along in the sequential evaluation process based on "residual functional capacity," or functional limitations resulting from their medical impairments. The Listings are organized into 14 body systems for adults and 15 body systems for children. Special senses-related disorders that affect the ability to hear are evaluated under SSA Listings 2.00 for adults and Listings 102.00 for children. SSA organizes the evaluation of hearing loss into two broad categories: hearing loss not treated with cochlear implantation and hearing loss treated with cochlear implantation. The focus of this report is hearing loss in adults and children treated with cochlear implantation.

The current Listings that address hearing loss treated with cochlear implantation (2.11 and 102.11) contain criteria that evaluate hearing ability through a word recognition score determined using the Hearing in Noise Test (HINT) performed in a quiet sound field. To be used in SSA's program, HINT testing must be performed on a person with properly functioning cochlear implants set at normal settings, with no visual testing cues, in a quiet sound field and at 60 dB HL (decibels in hearing level). SSA seeks to generalize the Listings criteria found in 2.11B and 102.11B (of Subpart P of Part 404, *Listing of Impairments*) so that the criteria can be evaluated with the results from hearing tests other than the HINT but with similar levels of validity, specificity, sensitivity, and reliability. Unlike the Listing for hearing loss in individuals with cochlear implants, the Listing for hearing loss *not* treated with cochlear implantation (2.10 and 102.10) does not specify a test (i.e., the HINT). Instead, it requires a "word recognition score of 40 percent or less in the better ear determined using a standardized list of phonetically balanced monosyllabic words."

STATEMENT OF TASK

SSA has requested that a consensus committee of the National Academies of Sciences, Engineering, and Medicine identify and recommend generalized testing procedures and criteria for evaluating the level of functional hearing ability needed to make a disability determination in adults and children after cochlear implantation. The committee will produce a report detailing and supporting their findings, conclusions, and recommendations based on published evidence (to the extent possible) and professional judgment (where published evidence is lacking). The committee will:

1. Identify and describe the salient test characteristics of the HINT, which is currently used to determine the functional hearing ability in adults or children with hearing loss treated with cochlear implantation, and provide recommendations as to how to generalize those characteristics into criteria that can be applied to other validated hearing tests for persons with cochlear implants.
2. Describe the characteristics of hearing tests, administered in the sound field, either binaurally or monaurally, in either quiet or noise, that are in use for those with cochlear implants, and describe to the degree possible:
    a. The availability of the selected tests with respect to the instruments themselves, trained administrators of the tests, and insurance coverage or costs incurred with testing;
    b. The patient burden of undergoing these tests;
    c. Whether testing procedures or parameters, or the appropriateness of the test itself, vary based on the age of the person being tested;
    d. Whether the test outcomes are expected to vary based on demographic or other patient characteristic factors, including repeated testing with the same instrument; and

e. The validity, specificity, sensitivity, reliability, and generalizability of the tests.
3. Among the hearing tests described in task 2, identify those with characteristics most similar to the HINT, determine which tests, performed in the sound field, either binaurally or monaurally, in either quiet or noise, produce measurements most closely analogous to the word recognition score of the HINT (given HINT testing parameters of properly functioning cochlear implants set at normal settings, with no visual testing cues, in a quiet sound field, at 60 dB HL), and describe to the degree possible:
   a. What differences exist between the identified tests and the HINT in terms of the specific elements of hearing ability they measure;
   b. The committee's recommendations as to how scores from the identified tests can be compared or converted to equivalent scores on the HINT; and
   c. The committee's recommendations for the scores on hearing tests that correspond to a level of functional hearing ability that causes marked and severe functional limitation in a child or that prevents an adult from doing any gainful activity, regardless of his or her age, education, or work experience, and whether those scores can be expressed in a form comparable between hearing tests such as percentile or standard deviation from the norm.
4. Examine the special considerations inherent in evaluating hearing ability in persons with single-sided deafness or asymmetric hearing loss receiving a cochlear implant and describe:
   a. Any special considerations in the testing and treatment of persons with bilateral but unequal hearing loss;
   b. Whether there is a correlation between the presence and degree of hearing loss in the less-affected ear and the recovery time or treatment for individuals with single-sided deafness or asymmetric hearing loss receiving a cochlear implant in their more-affected ear;
   c. Whether there is a level of hearing ability in the less-affected ear which would render cochlear implantation in the more-affected ear immaterial with respect to meeting the severity of hearing loss in the Listings (i.e., would not prevent an adult from engaging in any gainful activity nor a child from having "marked" limitations in two domains of functioning or an "extreme" limitation in one domain);
   d. Whether the tests identified in task 3 remain appropriate for testing hearing ability in persons with single-sided deafness

or asymmetric hearing loss receiving a cochlear implant and why, and if there are any differences in how the tests should be administered or interpreted; and

e. Whether the equivalent scores identified in task 3 remain accurate proxies for the HINT word recognition scores when assessing persons with single-sided deafness or asymmetric hearing loss receiving a cochlear implant.

In its discussion with SSA, the committee interpreted its charge to provide SSA with a recommendation for tests that would be accessible and feasible for widespread use by audiology clinics, and that would align with standard clinical practice.

COCHLEAR IMPLANTS

Cochlear implants are small electronic devices that help provide a sense of sound to profoundly deaf or severely hard-of-hearing individuals. They function differently from hearing aids, as implants do not amplify sounds to improve normal hearing; instead, they give a person a representation of sounds in the environment, which in turn helps with understanding speech. Cochlear implants are surgically implanted and work by replacing the function of the damaged cochlea (inner ear) and stimulating the auditory nerve directly. The most recently published data from the National Institute on Deafness and Other Communication Disorders state that in 2012 approximately 58,000 adults and 38,000 children in the United States were reported to have cochlear implants. However, due to the expansion of indications and implantations in the past decade, those numbers are now a significant under-estimate. The American Cochlear Implant Alliance estimates that there were a total of 217,000 cochlear implant users in the United States in 2019. That number is based on a 9 percent annual growth rate from 2012.

In early clinical trials, to qualify for cochlear implants, adults were required to score 0 percent on open-set measures of sentence recognition, and children were required to demonstrate bilateral profound sensorineural hearing loss, as the outcomes with cochlear implants were unknown. As the safety and efficacy of cochlear implants became known, the criteria to receive a cochlear implant changed. Traditionally, most devices based candidacy on a sentence score for adults and on a word score for children. However, in 2019 the U.S. Food and Drug Administration (FDA) approved the MED-EL devices for use in children (5 years of age and older) and adults with single-sided deafness (SSD) and asymmetric hearing loss (AHL). Both approvals include indications that base candidacy on a word score for both children and adults and represent a trend toward the use of monosyllabic word measures with both children and adults in the field of cochlear implants. From 2000 to early 2020, cochlear implants were FDA-approved for use in children beginning at 12 months of age; however, in March 2020, Cochlear Ltd. (Sydney, Australia) received FDA approval to expand the labeled indications from 12 to 9 months of age. For young children who are deaf or severely hard-of-hearing, using a cochlear implant exposes them to sounds during an optimal period for developing auditory speech and language skills. There is a growing body of literature demonstrating that children who receive cochlear implants before 12 months of age significantly outperform children who are implanted between 12 and 18 months on measures of language development, speech perception, and vocabulary as well as speech intelligibility (i.e., how well others are able to understand one's speech).

THE HEARING IN NOISE TEST

The HINT, first published in 1994, is the test that SSA currently uses to determine functional hearing ability in adults or children with hearing loss treated with cochlear implantation. The HINT measures sentence recognition and is standardized to be administered with background noise, although SSA uses the HINT sentences in a quiet sound field. The HINT corpus is composed of 250 sentences, which are categorized into 25 lists. The sentences for the HINT were adapted from 336 Bamford-Kowal-Bench (BKB) sentences written in British English to American English sentences of equivalent content and length. During the test, the subject uses both ears (binaural hearing) and is required to repeat sentences in a quiet environment and with competing noise presented from different directions.

The volume of each sentence is adjusted based on listener response. Following each correct response, the volume is decreased, which increases the level of difficulty for the next sentence on the list. After an incorrect response the volume is increased, which reduces the difficulty for hearing each subsequent sentence. The level of background noise is held constant.

The HINT was developed in 1994 to be adaptively measured (i.e., the signal-to-noise ratio was adjusted between trials according to whether the response was correct) in order to minimize floor and ceiling effects.[1] However, clinical use of the HINT does not incorporate adaptive administration; rather, the sentences are typically presented at a fixed level "in quiet," that is, in a quiet environment. This, along with improvements in cochlear implant technology, has resulted in individuals with cochlear implants scoring consistently near the ceiling on the HINT. Unilateral cochlear implant

---

[1] A ceiling effect occurs when the items on a test are so easy that most people would achieve or be close to the highest possible score.

recipients with post-lingual onset of deafness are routinely achieving 60 percent open-set word recognition, on average. Indeed, an increasingly higher proportion of adult and pediatric cochlear implant recipients demonstrate at or near ceiling-level performance for sentence recognition in quiet.

Despite its common inclusion in cochlear implant candidacy and outcomes criteria for cochlear implant recipients, recent work has demonstrated that the HINT is limited not just by its ceiling effects when presented in quiet or fixed signal-to-noise ratios, but also by its administration, its ecologic validity, and its availability.

In particular, the lack of availability of the HINT materials has created various problems. When the Minimum Speech Test Battery (MSTB) was first conceptualized in 1996, cochlear implant surgery was performed only at select major medical centers in the United States. Those centers were able to obtain necessary test materials and had the appropriate equipment set up to perform speech performance assessments. However, due to the HINT's exclusion from the most recent MSTB and because it is no longer available for purchase, the HINT is difficult for clinics across the United States to obtain.

As requested in the Statement of Task, the committee describes salient characteristics of the HINT. A summary is provided below in Table S-1.

CHARACTERISTICS OF SELECTED SENTENCE AND WORD TESTS

Chapter 4 provides an overview of characteristics of selected speech tests that are commonly used to evaluate hearing loss in adults and children with cochlear implants, in addition to the HINT. Table S-2 briefly summarizes those tests and their reliability or other salient characteristics. With the exception of the HINT and the Digit Triplet test, the tests presented in Table S-2 are readily available for purchase in the United States.

TESTING HEARING ABILITY IN PERSONS WITH SINGLE-SIDED DEAFNESS OR ASYMMETRIC HEARING LOSS RECEIVING A COCHLEAR IMPLANT

Historically, indications to qualify for a cochlear implant and indications to qualify for disability due to hearing loss have required patients to have significant *bilateral* hearing loss. With cochlear implants, this was a decision made in early clinical trials when the safety and efficacy of cochlear implants were not yet proven. The decision to provide cochlear implants to patients with significant SSD or AHL was made only recently in 2019,

TABLE S-1 Salient Characteristics of the Hearing in Noise Test (HINT)

Characteristic	Description
Sentences	The HINT is composed of 250 sentences that are divided into 25 lists
Adaptive assessment	The original design of the assessment uses an adaptive procedure to adjust the speech level to prevent ceiling effects[a]
Intelligibility of materials	Phonemic content and word familiar based on American English are balanced across 25 lists of 10 sentences
Accessibility across multiple languages	Translated into at least 11 languages[b]
Speech-spectrum noise	Noise is spectrally matched to the amplitude and frequency response of the recorded sentences
Recorded speech by singular speaker	The HINT materials were recorded by a singular male speaker
Co-located speech and noise signals	Assessment designed presentation from a singular sound source (i.e., speech and noise come from the same speaker)
Quick assessment tool	Each sentence list from the HINT takes approximately 2 minutes to complete
Material access	At this time, the HINT is difficult to obtain outside of large academic medical centers

[a] The intended use may not be consistent with actual use due to fixed-presentation recommendations from the Minimum Speech Test Battery in 1996.

[b] The clinician presenting the materials must be fluent in the language of administration.

when FDA approved cochlear implants for adults and children (ages 5 and up) with SSD and AHL. This decision was based on research demonstrating that most individuals with SSD or AHL demonstrated improvements in word and sentence recognition in quiet in the implanted ear, improvements in sentence recognition in noise when noise was presented to the better hearing ear, improvements in sound localization, and improvements in self-perceived quality of hearing.

The presence of bilateral profound hearing loss not treated with a cochlear implant will prevent adults from engaging in any gainful activity and will result in children having marked limitations in various domains of functioning. Currently, adult patients without a cochlear implant meet the criteria in the Listings if they demonstrate an average air conduction hearing threshold of 90 dB or greater in the better ear and an average bone conduction hearing threshold of 60 dB or greater in the better ear (2.10A), or if they demonstrate a word recognition score of 40 percent correct or

TABLE S-2 Reliability and Other Notable Characteristics of Selected Sentence and Word Tests

Test	Year of Publication	Target Population	Reliability and Other Notable Characteristics
Sentence Tests			
Central Institute for the Deaf (CID) Sentences	1955	Adults	Low reliability: individual test lists do not produce equivalent scores.
City University of New York (CUNY) Sentences	1985	Adults	Sentence lists are of equivalent difficulty.
Hearing in Noise Test (HINT)	1994	Adults	Use of one test list is capable of detecting differences in reception thresholds for sentences of 2.98 decibels (dB) in quiet and 2.41 dB in noise. Confidence intervals improve as the number of sentence lists increases. When used with listeners with hearing loss, reliability is quite close to that demonstrated for listeners with normal hearing. Note: This reliability information is for results obtained with the HINT administered as intended by the test authors. Use of the HINT with cochlear implant users almost always deviates from these procedures. Availability is limited as the test is no longer sold.
HINT-Children (HINT-C)	1996	Children	Reliability is similar to that of the HINT. Younger children (i.e., 6–12 years of age) perform significantly poorer than older children and adults. Availability is limited as the test is no longer sold.
Quick Speech in Noise Test (QuickSIN)	2004	Adults	Each of the test's 12 lists produce equivalent scores. A single list is accurate to +/− 2.2. dB (80% confidence interval) and to +/− 2.7 dB (95% confidence interval). Reliability improves as the number of lists administered increases.
Bamford-Kowal-Bench Speech in Noise (BKB-SIN) Test	2005	Children and cochlear implant candidates and users	Reliability of the BKB-SIN is related to the number of test items, age, and cochlear implant use. Largest gains in reliability are obtained with a move from administration of one list to two lists.

TABLE S-2 Continued

Test	Year of Publication	Target Population	Reliability and Other Notable Characteristics
Arizona Biomedical (AzBio) Sentences Test	2005	Adults	The 15 lists of sentences available in the AzBio test produce equivalent results.
Pediatric Arizona Biomedical (AzBio) Sentences Test	2014	Children	The AzBio test lists produce equivalent scores. Confidence intervals are provided for administration of one and two sentence lists per test condition and are based on the methods of Thornton and Raffin (1978).
Phonetically-Balanced Kindergarten (PBK) Words	1949	Children	Of the original four PBK sentences lists, Lists 1, 3, and 4 have been found to be equivalent. These are the lists used in clinical practice.
Word Tests			
Northwestern University Test No. 6 (NU-6) Words	1966	Adults	Testing with listeners with normal hearing and listeners with hearing loss have revealed good inter-list equivalence and high test–retest reliability.
Maryland CNC Words	1984	Adults	The test offers six equivalent and reliable lists.
Lexical Neighborhood Test (LNT)	1995	Children	High reliability on the LNT and the MLNT has been demonstrated in excellent test–retest reliability and strong correlations between test sessions. The tests' matched lists provide equivalent performance.
Multisyllabic Neighborhood Test (MLNT)	1995	Children	
Words in Noise Test (WIN)	2003	Adults	The WIN is sensitive to the presence of hearing loss, even just high-frequency hearing loss. A signal-to-babble ratio greater than 6 dB on this test is an abnormal finding.
Digit Triplet	2004	Adults	This test uses numerical digits rather than words. It is a highly reliable test as evidenced by a measurement error of less than 1 dB. Reliability is equivalent for tests administered in audiology clinics as well as in private homes. Availability in the United States is unknown.

less in the better ear determined using a standardized list of phonetically balanced monosyllabic words (2.10B). Thus, patients' hearing loss must be bilateral and must have a significant impact on their ability to communicate. If an adult patient's hearing loss has been treated with a cochlear implant, he/she is considered disabled for 1 year after initial implantation (2.11A). On occasion, adults and children will continue to demonstrate difficulty hearing even after they receive a cochlear implant. When this occurs, they can still qualify for disability if they demonstrate a word recognition score of 60 percent correct or less determined using the HINT Sentences test (2.11B, 102.11). Most adults and children with bilateral significant hearing loss who receive a cochlear implant derive benefit from the device, and the improvements they receive often prevent them from qualifying for disability after 1 year of using the device.

As indicated previously, cochlear implants were not yet approved by FDA for use in patients with SSD or AHL when the current SSA guidelines were developed. Prior to approval of cochlear implants for SSD and AHL, indications for cochlear implants, like indications for disability, were based on the "best" hearing situation. Thus, most cochlear implant recipients who were implanted previously qualified for disability under both 2.10 and 2.11 prior to receiving a cochlear implant as they likely experienced significant hearing loss in each ear. *That would not be the case for patients who currently receive a cochlear implant due to SSD or AHL because they possess normal or near-normal hearing in their better ear.*

Under current SSA guidelines, patients with SSD or AHL automatically qualify for disability for a period of 1 year following cochlear implantation, with no consideration given to the hearing in their better ear. To remain consistent with the wording and rationale used in current guidelines for hearing loss not treated with cochlear implantation (Listings 2.10 and 102.10), it is reasonable to consider the hearing in the better ear when determining whether a patient with a cochlear implant qualifies for disability due to hearing loss after he/she receives a cochlear implant.

CONCLUSIONS AND RECOMMENDATIONS

Since its development in 1994, the HINT has been widely used to measure cochlear implant candidacy and post-operative outcomes. However, the test characteristics, the state of cochlear implant technology, and the environment that made the HINT a common choice of assessment in 1994 are different in 2021. The HINT has several limitations in its characteristics and deviation from its intended use. The MSTB recommendations note that "advances in technology, improvements in outcomes, and changes in candidacy criteria have resulted in ceiling effects on the HINT sentences when presented in quiet." FDA usage in effectiveness studies and unclear candidacy criteria from insurance providers (e.g., the Centers for Medicare & Medicaid Services) add to the limitations of the test. Finally, due to its exclusion from the most recent MSTB and the fact that it is no longer available for purchase, the HINT is difficult for clinics across the United States to obtain.

More recently, word recognition testing—which includes the administration of a phonemically balanced word list such as the Northwestern University Auditory Test Number 6, Central Institute for the Deaf W-22, or the Maryland consonant–nucleus–consonant word lists—has come to be employed in most audiology clinics. Monosyllabic word recognition is also currently the standard for pediatric cochlear implant candidacy, and the field is moving toward use of a monosyllabic word recognition criterion for determining adult candidacy in the United States. Additionally, for more than two decades monosyllabic word recognition has been used to characterize post-operative outcomes for both adult and pediatric cochlear implant recipients. Furthermore, SSA has been using monosyllabic words to determine initial and continued eligibility for SSA benefits for individuals with hearing loss who have not been treated with cochlear implantation.

The committee was tasked with recommending how scores from the identified tests can be compared with or converted to equivalent scores on the HINT. However, given the committee's concerns with the utility of the HINT and limitations such as ceiling effects and lack of availability, deriving equivalent scores on the HINT would produce scores with limited interpretability. Additionally, while it may be of value to have a common metric or a conversion equivalent in the presence of newer tests, this task is complicated by a lack of large research studies with head-to-head comparisons of the HINT to other tests. Thus, the committee was unable to calculate meaningful equivalent test scores for the HINT.

The current use of the HINT sentences as criteria for cochlear implantation likely suffers from ceiling effects of the test materials, given improvements in modern cochlear implant technology and a lack of availability of test materials. Research may support an update of assessment of cochlear implementation via different materials. Speech assessment via sentences fundamentally differs from assessment via individual words because it offers context to the information, and such context may result in improved scores in speech understanding. Thus, given the difficulty of obtaining the HINT, the shift in the cochlear implant community toward using word tests, and the fact that SSA already uses word tests for individuals with hearing loss who do not have a cochlear implant, the committee makes the following recommendation:

Given the limitations of the Hearing in Noise Test, the committee recommends the use of a monosyllabic word recognition test to assess hearing loss in individuals treated with cochlear implantation, consistent with what the U.S. Social Security Administration currently uses to determine disability in adults and children with hearing loss not treated with cochlear implantation. The administration of the word test should include a full word list that is standardized and phonetically or phonemically balanced.

As of this writing, examples of tests that meet those criteria and that are commonly used by audiologists to evaluate hearing loss in people with cochlear implants include the consonant–nucleus–consonant words or the Northwestern University Test No. 6 for adults and the Phonetically Balanced Kindergarten or Lexical Neighborhood Test for children.

SSA also asked the committee whether the tests identified in task 3 remain appropriate for testing hearing ability in persons with single-sided deafness or asymmetric hearing loss receiving a cochlear implant and why, and if there are any differences in how the tests should be administered or interpreted. The committee notes that the same tests and testing parameters can be used, with a few additional considerations. Testing for disability for hearing loss has typically focused on the test results obtained with the better ear. Thus, a patient who receives a cochlear implant due to SSD or AHL should be required to participate in testing that represents the listening situation that he/she uses on a daily basis, which typically includes an un-occluded better ear and an ear using hearing technology. Alternatively, it could be based on the individual being required to meet current requirements for hearing loss not treated with cochlear implantation in the ear not treated with a cochlear implant (Listing 2.10 and 102.10).

The Statement of Task requests that the committee "identify and recommend generalized testing procedures and criteria for evaluating the level of functional hearing ability needed to make a disability determination in adults and children after cochlear implantation." Thus, based on standard clinical practice and the committee's professional judgment:

> The committee recommends using the following presentation level and standardized test setup:
> - 60 decibel sound pressure level using hearing technology recommended for the individual that is functioning properly and adjusted to the individual's normal settings. In cases of single-sided deafness or asymmetric hearing loss, the non-implanted ear should not be occluded for testing,
> - The level should be calibrated for sound field presentation,

- The test material should be recorded to ensure standardized administration,
- Testing should occur in quiet in a sound-treated booth, and
- The listener should be seated 1 meter from the loudspeaker at 0° azimuth.

Finally, the Statement of Task asks the committee

for the scores on hearing tests that correspond to a level of functional hearing ability that causes marked and severe functional limitation in a child or that prevents an adult from doing any gainful activity, regardless of his or her age, education, or work experience and whether those scores can be expressed in a form comparable between hearing tests such as percentile or standard deviation from the norm.

In response, the committee suggests that SSA use the same cut-off criteria for evaluating hearing loss in individuals with cochlear implants as the current Listing for hearing loss in individuals without cochlear implants. That cut-off aligns with the criteria used in the most recent FDA clinical trials for cochlear implants. Specifically, FDA trials use a cut-off score of 40 percent correct or less in the ear to be implanted and 50 percent correct or less in the contralateral ear on a recorded monosyllabic word test presented at 60 A-weighted dB (dB A).

The committee recommends a score of 40 percent correct or less on a monosyllabic word test as the cut-off criterion for hearing loss in adults and children treated with cochlear implantation, consistent with the current U.S. Social Security Administration criterion for adults and children with hearing loss not treated with cochlear implantation.

The committee's recommendation would allow SSA to provide a singular speech recognition measure and criterion across all individuals, irrespective of hearing technology. Given that cochlear implants are currently the final step on the hearing health care continuum, the committee believes that should an individual with a cochlear implant continue to meet the criteria for cochlear implantation after they have been implanted with their device, they clearly have demonstrated that the cochlear implant has not provided significant benefit. As such, the cochlear implant recipient most likely has a disability related to hearing loss.

No single test can fully capture the broad neurological faculties that allow for speech and language understanding. Speech perception tests assess a diverse set of abilities, and each provides different insight into specific auditory and processing capabilities. As a single measure, monosyllabic word tests cannot capture the full auditory and communication profile of a listener, but the committee believes that it is a good proxy. The use of monosyllabic words does not penalize or reward a listener for being adept at top-down processing. Furthermore, the use of monosyllabic words is consistent with current clinical speech audiometry practice and is readily accessible. While it was not within the committee's scope of work, the committee notes as a consideration that additional information from self-report or parent-report questionnaires may be useful in better characterizing an individual's real-world communicative functioning. To fully evaluate auditory function, it can be helpful to include a subjective perspective from the patient or from their parent. Self-report or parent-report measurements, when used as a supplement to auditory threshold and speech testing, can help capture the complete picture of the impact of hearing loss in a given individual.

As a final note, the above recommendations were made based on the state of knowledge available to committee members at the time of writing. As advances in clinical practice, assessment measures, and hearing technology emerge, it is possible that better measures for assessing significant disability will become available. Therefore, should more information become known in the future, it may be necessary to revisit the recommendations in this report.

1

Introduction

The U.S. Social Security Administration (SSA) administers the Social Security Disability Insurance program (Title II of the Social Security Act) and the Supplemental Security Income (SSI) program (Title XVI of the Social Security Act). Title II pays disability benefits to people who are "insured" under the Act. The benefits are paid out of the Social Security trust fund, which is funded by the Social Security tax on individuals' earnings. The Act also provides benefits to certain disabled dependents of insured individuals. Title XVI provides SSI payments to adults and children (under age 18) who are disabled and have limited income and resources.

When SSA evaluates disability claims based on a physical or mental impairment, it requires sufficient evidence to (1) establish the presence of a medically determinable physical or mental impairment(s), (2) assess the degree of functional limitation the impairment(s) imposes, and (3) project the probable duration of the impairment(s). Once SSA establishes the presence of a severe medically determinable physical or mental impairment(s), it determines whether the impairment(s) meets or medically equals (i.e., is equivalent in severity to) the criteria in the *Listing of Impairments* (the Listings), which are lists of medical conditions that qualify a candidate for disability benefits regardless of the applicant's age, education, or work experience. The Listings are organized into 14 body systems for adults and 15 body systems for children. Each of the Listings includes impairments that, for adults, SSA considers severe enough to prevent any gainful activity and, for children, SSA considers severe enough to cause marked and severe functional limitations. If an individual does not meet Listings-level criteria, they can still qualify for disability further along in the sequential evaluation process based on "residual functional capacity," or functional limitations resulting from their medical impairments.

Special senses-related disorders that affect the ability to hear are evaluated under Listing 2.00 for adults and Listing 102.00 for children. SSA organizes the evaluation of hearing loss into two broad categories: hearing loss not treated with cochlear implantation and hearing loss treated with cochlear implantation.

The focus of this report is adults and children with cochlear implantation. In a *Federal Register* notice (Vol. 75, No. 105) published on June 2, 2010, SSA described in its rules and regulations the type of audiometric testing that is needed for those with cochlear implantation to be considered disabled until age 5 or for 1 year after implantation, whichever is later:

> After that period, we [SSA] need word recognition testing performed with any age-appropriate version of the Hearing in Noise Test (HINT) or the Hearing in Noise Test for Children (HINT-C) to determine whether your impairment meets 102.11B. This testing must be conducted in quiet in a sound field. Your implant must be functioning properly and adjusted to your normal settings. The sentences should be presented at 60 dB HL (Hearing Level) and without any visual cues.

The current Listings that address hearing loss treated with cochlear implantation (2.11 and 102.11) contain criteria that evaluate hearing ability through a word recognition score determined using the Hearing in Noise Test (HINT) performed in a quiet sound field. To be used in SSA's program, HINT testing must be performed on a person with properly functioning cochlear implants set at normal settings, with no visual testing cues, in a quiet sound field, and at 60 dB HL (decibel hearing level).[1]

Unlike the Listing for hearing loss in individuals with cochlear implants, the Listing for hearing loss not treated with cochlear implantation (2.10 and 102.10) does not specify a test (i.e., the HINT). Instead, it requires a "word recognition score of 40 percent or less in the better ear determined using a standardized list of phonetically balanced monosyllabic words."

SSA seeks to generalize the listing criteria found in 2.11B and 102.11B (of Subpart P of Part 404, *Listing of Impairments*), the Listings for hearing loss treated with cochlear implantation, so that they can be evaluated with the results from hearing tests other than the HINT while maintaining similar levels of validity, specificity, sensitivity, and reliability.

---

[1] dB HL = decibels in hearing level, the decibel measure displayed on an audiometer, normalized so that 0 dB HL = average normal for all frequencies.

INTRODUCTION

STATEMENT OF TASK

SSA requested that a consensus committee of the National Academies of Sciences, Engineering, and Medicine identify and recommend generalized testing procedures and criteria for evaluating the level of functional hearing ability needed to make a disability determination in adults and children after cochlear implantation. The committee will produce a report detailing and supporting their findings, conclusions, and recommendations based on published evidence (to the extent possible) and professional judgment (where published evidence is lacking). The committee will:

1. Identify and describe the salient test characteristics of the HINT, which is currently used to determine the functional hearing ability in adults or children with hearing loss treated with cochlear implantation, and provide recommendations as to how to generalize those characteristics into criteria that can be applied to other validated hearing tests for persons with cochlear implants.
2. Describe the characteristics of hearing tests, administered in the sound field, either binaurally or monaurally, in either quiet or noise, that are in use for those with cochlear implants, and describe to the degree possible:
   a. The availability of the selected tests with respect to the instruments themselves, trained administrators of the tests, and insurance coverage or costs incurred with testing;
   b. The patient burden of undergoing these tests;
   c. Whether testing procedures or parameters, or the appropriateness of the test itself, vary based on the age of the person being tested;
   d. Whether the test outcomes are expected to vary based on demographic or other patient characteristic factors, including repeated testing with the same instrument; and
   e. The validity, specificity, sensitivity, reliability, and generalizability of the tests.
3. Among the hearing tests described in task 2, identify those with characteristics most similar to the HINT, determine which tests, performed in the sound field, either binaurally or monaurally, in either quiet or noise, produce measurements most closely analogous to the word recognition score of the HINT (given HINT testing parameters of properly functioning cochlear implants set at normal settings, with no visual testing cues, in a quiet sound field, at 60 dB HL), and describe to the degree possible:

a. What differences exist between the identified tests and the HINT in terms of the specific elements of hearing ability they measure;
b. The committee's recommendations as to how scores from the identified tests can be compared or converted to equivalent scores on the HINT; and
c. The committee's recommendations for the scores on hearing tests that correspond to a level of functional hearing ability that causes marked and severe functional limitation in a child or that prevents an adult from doing any gainful activity, regardless of his or her age, education, or work experience, and whether those scores can be expressed in a form comparable between hearing tests such as percentile or standard deviation from the norm.
4. Examine the special considerations inherent in evaluating hearing ability in persons with single-sided deafness or asymmetric hearing loss receiving a cochlear implant and describe:
   a. Any special considerations in the testing and treatment of persons with bilateral but unequal hearing loss;
   b. Whether there is a correlation between the presence and degree of hearing loss in the less-affected ear and the recovery time or treatment for individuals with single-sided deafness or asymmetric hearing loss receiving a cochlear implant in their more-affected ear;
   c. Whether there is a level of hearing ability in the less-affected ear which would render cochlear implantation in the more-affected ear immaterial with respect to meeting the severity of hearing loss in the Listings (i.e., would not prevent an adult from engaging in any gainful activity nor a child from having "marked" limitations in two domains of functioning or an "extreme" limitation in one domain[2]);
   d. Whether the tests identified in task 3 remain appropriate for testing hearing ability in persons with single-sided deafness or asymmetric hearing loss receiving a cochlear implant and why, and if there are any differences in how the tests should be administered or interpreted; and
   e. Whether the equivalent scores identified in task 3 remain accurate proxies for the HINT word recognition scores when assessing persons with single-sided deafness or asymmetric hearing loss receiving a cochlear implant.

---

[2] See 20 Code of Federal Regulations 416.926a and DI (disability insurance) 25225.030, DI 25225.035, DI 25225.040, DI 25225.045, DI 25225.050, and DI 25225.055.

APPROACH TO THE TASK

The National Academies assembled a committee of experts to address the task. Members with diverse backgrounds and expertise were appointed to focus on the different aspects of the task. Specifically, the members have expertise in audiology, otolaryngology, cochlear implantation in both children and adults, hearing loss testing, biostatistics, and epidemiology.

The committee met four times. It sponsored one open meeting, which enabled SSA representatives and the committee members to interact directly and to discuss the committee's charge. In its discussion with SSA, the committee interpreted its charge to provide SSA with a recommendation for tests that would be accessible and feasible for widespread use by audiology clinics. Furthermore, that guiding principle led the committee to search for tests that would align with standard clinical practice.

In support of the committee's discussions and deliberations, the committee instructed the staff to conduct targeted literature searches and to gather information from relevant texts, scientific journals and professional societies, and federal sources.

The review began with a search of online databases for U.S. and international English-language literature from 2010 through 2020. This search covered PubMed and Scopus as well as SSA and the National Academies Press websites. The search terms used included the names of the hearing tests the committee members identified intersected with key words from each of the questions in the Statement of Task. Staff initially reviewed more than 1,132 titles and abstracts, which the committee members carefully reviewed for relevance to the committee's task. Committee members and project staff identified additional literature as needed throughout the course of the study to supplement the initial search, using systematic reviews when available.

COCHLEAR IMPLANTS

Cochlear implants are small electronic devices that help provide a sense of sound to profoundly deaf or severely hard-of-hearing individuals. They function differently from hearing aids, as implants do not amplify sounds to improve normal hearing; instead they give a person a representation of sounds in the environment, which in turn helps with understanding speech (NIDCD, 2017). Cochlear implants are surgically implanted and work by replacing the function of the damaged cochlea (inner ear) and stimulating the auditory nerve directly. The most recently published data state that in 2012 approximately 58,000 adults and 38,000 children had cochlear implants in the United States (NIDCD, 2017). Due to expansion of indications and implantation in the past decade, these numbers are now a significant under-estimate. The American Cochlear Implant Alliance estimates that there were a total of 217,000 cochlear implant users in the United States in 2019. That estimate was based on a 9 percent annual growth rate from 2012 (ACIA, 2021).

Adults who lose some or most of their hearing as they age frequently benefit from cochlear implants, as they learn to associate the signals from the implant with sounds they remember, including speech, without requiring visual cues such as those provided by lipreading or sign language. For infants and young children without additional disabilities, cochlear implants placed early afford a child the ability to communicate via listening and spoken language at levels comparable to those of their same-age peers with typical hearing (Mayo Clinic, 2020; Niparko et al., 2010).

In early clinical trials, to qualify for cochlear implants, adults were required to score 0 percent on open-set measures of sentence recognition[3] (Waltzman and Shapiro, 1999), and children were required to demonstrate bilateral profound sensorineural hearing loss, as the outcomes with cochlear implants were not known. As the safety and efficacy of cochlear implants became known, the criteria to receive a cochlear implant changed. Currently, three different manufacturers produce cochlear implants that have received U.S. Food and Drug Administration (FDA) approval in the United States. The approved indications for those devices vary depending on the timing of the approval and the stated goals of the clinical trial used to obtain FDA approval. Traditionally, most devices based candidacy on a sentence score for adults and on a word score for children. In 2013 and 2014 FDA approved two devices that used acoustic and electric hearing for rehabilitation (the Nucleus Hybrid Implant System and the MED-EL electric-acoustic stimulation, respectively). For each device candidacy was based on more lenient audiometric test results and on an aided word recognition score and not on a sentence score. In 2017 FDA approved the clinical trial to evaluate the Nucleus CI532 cochlear implant in adults (NCT03007472). In that trial, adults were considered to be candidates for this device if they obtained a test score of 40 percent correct or less in the ear to be implanted and 50 percent correct or less in the contralateral ear on a recorded monosyllabic word test presented at 60 dB sound pressure level (SPL), with A weighting (NLM, 2020). In 2019 FDA approved the MED-EL system for use in children (5 years of age and older) and adults with single-sided deafness and asymmetric hearing loss. Both approvals include indications that base candidacy for cochlear implantation on a word score for both children and adults, and represent a trend toward the

---

[3] Open-set tasks are designed without limitations on the possible responses, such as an essay question on an exam or a speech recognition task for which the listener must provide a response without prompts.

INTRODUCTION

use of monosyllabic word measures with both children and adults in the field of cochlear implants.

Cochlear implants work by bypassing the damaged areas of the ear and directly stimulating the auditory nerve. Signals generated by the implant are transmitted by way of the auditory nerve to the brain, which interprets the signals as sound (NIDCD, 2017). The implant consists of an external part that is located behind the ear and an additional part that is surgically placed under the skin (see Figure 1-1). An implant consists of the following parts:

- A microphone, which picks up sounds from the environment.
- A speech processor, which selects and arranges sounds picked up by the microphone.
- A transmitter and receiver/stimulator, which receives signals from the speech processor and converts them into electric impulses.
- An electrode array, which collects the impulses from the stimulator and sends them to different regions of the auditory nerve.

The internal part of the implant is placed under the skin behind the ear during outpatient surgery. A thin wire and small electrodes lead to the cochlea (part of the inner ear). The wire sends signals to the vestibulocochlear

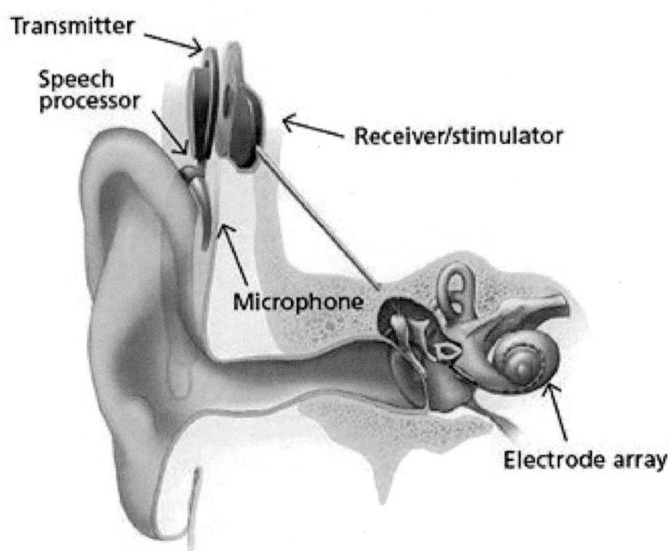

FIGURE 1-1 Diagram of an ear with a cochlear implant.
SOURCE: NIDCD, 2017.

nerve, which sends sound information to the brain to produce a hearing sensation. Although normal hearing is not restored, with appropriate therapy and practice the improved hearing experience can provide increased awareness of sounds in the environment as well as better communication through easier lipreading and listening (NIDCD, 2017).

Two recent literature reviews of post-implant performance were conducted by Boisvert et al. (2020) and by Buchman et al. (2020). Boisvert et al. (2020) reviewed 201 articles and reported that the average word recognition ability of implant recipients improved from 8.2 percent pre-implant to 53.9 percent post-implant and that 82 percent of post-lingually deafened adults and 53.4 percent of pre-lingually deafened adults demonstrated improvements of 15 percentage points or more. Buchman et al. (2020) reviewed 74 articles and identified 20 evidence-based consensus statements about cochlear implants, including

> Cochlear implants significantly improve speech recognition in both quiet and moderate noise in adults with severe, profound, or moderate sloping to profound bilateral sensorineural hearing loss; these gains in speech recognition are likely to remain stable over time. (p. 947)

From 2000 to early 2020 cochlear implants were FDA-approved for use in children beginning at 12 months of age; in March 2020, Cochlear Ltd. (Sydney, Australia) received FDA approval to expand the labeled indications from 12 months to 9 months of age (FDA, 2020). For young children who are deaf or severely hard-of-hearing, using a cochlear implant exposes them to sounds during an optimal period in which to develop speech and language skills (NIDCD, 2017).

According to the National Institutes of Health, research has shown that children who receive a cochlear implant followed by intensive therapy from about 12–18 months of age are better able to hear and comprehend sound and music and to use spoken language than children who receive implants when they are older. Studies have also shown that many eligible children who receive a cochlear implant by 12–18 months of age develop language skills at a rate comparable to children with normal hearing and that many succeed in mainstream classrooms (FDA, 2018).

There is a growing body of literature demonstrating that children who receive cochlear implants before 12 months of age significantly outperform children implanted between 12 and 18 months on measures of language development (Bergeson et al., 2010; Dettman et al., 2016; Houston and Miyamoto, 2010; Houston et al., 2012a,b; Tobey et al., 2013), speech perception (Holman et al., 2013; Tajudeen et al., 2010), vocabulary (Hayes et al., 2009; Houston and Miyamoto, 2010; Tomblin et al., 2005), and speech intelligibility (i.e., how well others are able to understand one's speech) (Habib et al., 2010). The likely reason is that the typically developing infant undergoes significant auditory and language development in the first year of life—all of which may be missed or delayed for infants with severe-to-profound hearing loss. For example, by 6 months of age infants are linking sound patterns with meanings, including events ("bye-bye"), persons ("mommy"), and familiar objects ("nose") (e.g., Bergelson and Swingley, 2012; Tincoff and Jusczyk, 1999, 2012). Word segmentation—the process by which a listener extracts meaningful units, such as individual words, from connected discourse—develops rapidly between 7.5 and 10.5 months (e.g., Jusczyk, 2002). By 8 months of age, infants exhibit long-term memory for newly acquired words, which is an important prerequisite for auditory-based language learning (Houston and Jusczyk, 2003; Jusczyk and Hohne, 1997).

Babies are exposed to multisensory stimuli shaping their auditory and language development with consistent auditory exposure to speech, music, and environmental sounds. Those auditory experiences are particularly influential during an infant's waking hours; however, infants with severe-to-profound hearing loss experience auditory deprivation prior to initial hearing aid fitting and typically wear their hearing aids for less than 4 hours per day in the first year of life (Walker et al., 2015). Consequently, infants with severe-to-profound sensorineural hearing loss, for whom auditory access audibility is limited, are deprived of critical auditory-based, language-learning opportunities prior to cochlear implantation (Levine et al., 2016).

INTRODUCTION TO THE HEARING IN NOISE TEST

The HINT, first published in 1994, is the test that SSA currently uses to determine functional hearing ability in adults or children with hearing loss who have been treated with cochlear implantation. The HINT measures sentence recognition and is standardized to be administered with background noise, although SSA uses the HINT sentences in a quiet sound field. The HINT corpus is composed of 250 sentences, which are categorized into 25 lists. The sentences for the HINT were adapted from 336 Bamford-Kowal-Bench (BKB) sentences written in British English (Bench et al., 1979) to American English sentences of equivalent content and length (Starkey Research, 2020). During the test the subject uses both ears (binaural hearing) and is required to repeat sentences in a quiet environment and with competing noise presented from different directions (California Ear Institute, 2020).

The volume of each sentence is adjusted based on listener response. Following each correct response, the volume is decreased, which increases the level of difficulty for the next sentence on the list. Conversely, the volume of the sentence is increased after each incorrect response, which reduces the difficulty for hearing each subsequent sentence. However, the level of background noise is held constant.

The HINT, as noted, was developed in 1994 to be adaptively measured (i.e., the signal-to-noise ratio was adjusted between trials according to whether the response was correct) in order to minimize floor and ceiling effects[4] (Nilsson et al., 1994). However, improvements in cochlear implant technology have resulted in individuals with cochlear implants scoring consistently near the ceiling on the HINT sentence test. Specifically, unilateral cochlear implant recipients with post-lingual onset of deafness are routinely achieving 60 percent open-set monosyllabic word recognition, on average, on the HINT (Buchman et al., 2020; Holden et al., 2013). Indeed, an increasingly higher proportion of adult and pediatric implant recipients demonstrate at or near ceiling-level performance for tests of sentence recognition in quiet (Dunn et al., 2020; Gifford et al., 2018).

ORGANIZATION OF THE REPORT

Chapter 2 is a primer on assessing speech perception, familiarizing the reader with terms, concepts, and considerations for speech recognition test presentation level setup. It defines numerous terms and introduces speech and word tests and highlights the distinctions between them. It also provides the background material necessary to understand items 1, 2, and 3c in the Statement of Task. Chapter 3 addresses the Statement of Task's item 1, which asks the committee to:

> *Identify and describe the salient test characteristics of the HINT, which is currently used to determine the functional hearing ability in adults or children with hearing loss treated with cochlear implantation, and provide recommendations as to how to generalize those characteristics into criteria that can be applied to other validated hearing tests for persons with cochlear implants.*

Chapter 4 describes the Statement of Task's item 2, that is,

> *Describe the characteristics of hearing tests, administered in the sound field, either binaurally or monaurally, in either quiet or noise, that are in use for those with cochlear implants, and describe to the degree possible, their availability, patient burden, the appropriateness of the test and whether test outcomes might vary based on demographic or other*

---

[4] The ceiling effect is observed when an independent variable no longer has an effect on a dependent variable or when the level above which variance in an independent variable is no longer measurable.

INTRODUCTION

patient characteristic factors, and the validity, specificity, sensitivity, reliability, and generalizability of the tests.

Chapter 5 addresses the Statement of Task's item 4, "examine special considerations in evaluating hearing ability in persons with single sided deafness or asymmetric hearing loss receiving a cochlear implant," and Chapter 6 addresses item 3:

Among the hearing tests described in task 2, identify those with characteristics most similar to the HINT, determine which tests, performed in the sound field, either binaurally or monaurally, in either quiet or noise, produce measurements most closely analogous to the word recognition score of the HINT.

A list of acronyms and abbreviations can be found at the beginning of the report.

REFERENCES

ACIA (American Cochlear Implant Alliance). 2021. *Cochlear implants: What is a cochlear implant?* https://www.acialliance.org/page/CochlearImplant (accessed January 15, 2021).

Bench, J., A. Kowal, and J. Bamford. 1979. The BKB (Bamford-Kowal-Bench) sentence lists for partially-hearing children. *British Journal of Audiology* 13(3):108–112.

Bergelson, E., and D. Swingley. 2012. At 6–9 months, human infants know the meanings of many common nouns. *Proceedings of the National Academy of Sciences* 109(9):3253–3258.

Bergeson, T. R., D. M. Houston, and R. T. Miyamoto. 2010. Effects of congenital hearing loss and cochlear implantation on audiovisual speech perception in infants and children. *Restorative Neurology and Neuroscience* 28(2):157–165.

Boisvert, I., M. Reis, A. Au, R. Cowan, and R. C. Dowell. 2020. Cochlear implantation outcomes in adults: A scoping review. *PLOS ONE* 15(5):e0232421.

Buchman, C. A., R. H. Gifford, D. S. Haynes, T. Lenarz, G. O'Donoghue, O. Adunka, A. Biever, R. J. Briggs, M. L. Carlson, P. Dai, C. L. Driscoll, H. W. Francis, B. J. Gantz, R. K. Gurgel, M. R. Hansen, M. Holcomb, E. Karltorp, M. Kirtane, J. Larky, E. A. M. Mylanus, J. Thomas Roland, Jr., S. R. Saeed, H. Skarzynski, P. H. Skarzynski, M. Syms, H. Teagle, P. H. van de Heyning, C. Vincent, H. Wu, T. Yamasoba, and T. Zwolan. 2020. Unilateral cochlear implants for severe, profound, or moderate sloping to profound bilateral sensorineural hearing loss: A systematic review and consensus statements. *JAMA Otolaryngology—Head & Neck Surgery* 146(10):942–953.

California Ear Institute. 2020. *Hearing in Noise Test (HINT)*. https://www.californiaearinstitute.com/audiology-services-hint-bay-area-ca.php (accessed October 17, 2020).

Dettman, S. J., R. C. Dowell, D. Choo, W. Arnott, Y. Abrahams, A. Davis, D. Dornan, J. Leigh, G. Constantinescu, R. Cowan, and R. J. Briggs. 2016. Long-term communication outcomes for children receiving cochlear implants younger than 12 months: A multicenter study. *Otology and Neurotology* 37(2):e82–e95.

Dunn, C. C., J. Oleson, A. Parkinson, M. R. Hansen, and B. J. Gantz. 2020. Nucleus Hybrid S12: Multicenter clinical trial results. *Laryngoscope* 130(10):E548–E558.

FDA (U.S. Food and Drug Administration). 2018. *What is a cochlear implant?* https://www.fda.gov/medical-devices/cochlear-implants/what-cochlear-implant (accessed October 17, 2020).

FDA. 2020. *"Off-label" and investigational use of marketed drugs, biologics, and medical devices.* https://www.fda.gov/regulatory-information/search-fda-guidance-documents/label-and-investigational-use-marketed-drugs-biologics-and-medical-devices (accessed September 24, 2020).

Gifford, R. H., L. Loiselle, S. Natale, S. W. Sheffield, L. W. Sunderhaus, M. S. Dietrich, and M. F. Dorman. 2018. Speech understanding in noise for adults with cochlear implants: Effects of hearing configuration, source location certainty, and head movement. *Journal of Speech, Language, and Hearing Research* 61(5):1306–1321.

Habib, M. G., S. B. Waltzman, B. Tajudeen, and M. A. Svirsky. 2010. Speech production intelligibility of early implanted pediatric cochlear implant users. *International Journal of Pediatric Otorhinolaryngology* 74(8):855–859.

Hayes, H., A. E. Geers, R. Treiman, and J. S. Moog. 2009. Receptive vocabulary development in deaf children with cochlear implants: Achievement in an intensive auditory–oral educational setting. *Ear and Hearing* 30(1):128–135.

Holden, L. K., C. Brenner, R. M. Reeder, and J. B. Firszt. 2013. Postlingual adult performance in noise with HiRes 120 and ClearVoice Low, Medium, and High. *Cochlear Implants International* 14(5):276–286.

Holman, M. A., M. L. Carlson, C. L. W. Driscoll, K. J. Grim, R. S. Petersson, D. P. Sladen, and R. P. Flick. 2013. Cochlear implantation in children 12 months of age and younger. *Otology and Neurotology* 34(2):251–258.

Houston, D. M., and P. W. Jusczyk. 2003. Infants' long-term memory for the sound patterns of words and voices. *Journal of Experimental Psychology: Human Perception and Performance* 29(6):1143–1154.

Houston, D. M., and R. T. Miyamoto. 2010. Effects of early auditory experience on word learning and speech perception in deaf children with cochlear implants: Implications for sensitive periods of language development. *Otology and Neurotology* 31(8):1248–1253.

Houston, D. M., J. Beer, T. R. Bergeson, S. B. Chin, D. B. Pisoni, and R. T. Miyamoto. 2012a. The ear is connected to the brain: Some new directions in the study of children with cochlear implants at Indiana University. *Journal of the American Academy of Audiology* 23(6):446–463.

Houston, D. M., J. Stewart, A. Moberly, G. Hollich, and R. T. Miyamoto. 2012b. Word learning in deaf children with cochlear implants: Effects of early auditory experience. *Developmental Science* 15(3):448–461.

Jusczyk, P. W. 2002. How infants adapt speech-processing capacities to native-language structure. *Current Directions in Psychological Science* 11(1):15–18.

Jusczyk, P. W., and E. A. Hohne. 1997. Infants' memory for spoken words. *Science* 277(5334):1984–1986.

Levine, D., K. Strother-Garcia, R. M. Golinkoff, and K. Hirsh-Pasek. 2016. Language development in the first year of life: What deaf children might be missing before cochlear implantation. *Otology and Neurotology* 37(2):e56–e62.

Mayo Clinic. 2020. *Cochlear implants.* https://www.mayoclinic.org/tests-procedures/cochlear-implants/about/pac-20385021 (accessed August 20, 2020).

NIDCD (National Institute on Deafness and Other Communication Disorders). 2017. *Cochlear implants.* https://www.nidcd.nih.gov/health/cochlear-implants (accessed August 19, 2020).

Nilsson, M., S. D. Soli, and J. A. Sullivan. 1994. Development of the Hearing in Noise Test for the measurement of speech reception thresholds in quiet and in noise. *Journal of the Acoustical Society of America* 95(2):1085–1099.

Niparko, J. K., E. A. Tobey, D. J. Thal, L. S. Eisenberg, N. Y. Wang, A. L. Quittner, and N. E. Fink. 2010. Spoken language development in children following cochlear implantation. *JAMA* 303(15):1498–1506.

NLM (National Library of Medicine). 2020. *Clinical evaluation of the Cochlear Nucleus CI532 cochlear implant in adults (SME).* https://www.clinicaltrials.gov/ct2/show/NCT03007472?term=NCT03007472&draw=2&rank=1 (accessed December 4, 2020).

Starkey Research. 2020. *The Hearing in Noise Test (HINT).* https://starkeypro.com/research/research-resources/hearing-in-noise-test.html (accessed October 17, 2020).

Tajudeen, B. A., S. B. Waltzman, D. Jethanamest, and M. A. Svirsky. 2010. Speech perception in congenitally deaf children receiving cochlear implants in the first year of life. *Otology and Neurotology* 31(8):1254–1260.

Tincoff, R., and P. W. Jusczyk. 1999. Some beginnings of word comprehension in 6-month-olds. *Psychological Science* 10(2):172–175.

Tincoff, R., and P. W. Jusczyk. 2012. Six-month-olds comprehend words that refer to parts of the body. *Infancy* 17(4):432–444.

Tobey, E. A., D. Thal, J. K. Niparko, L. S. Eisenberg, A. L. Quittner, and N. Y. Wang. 2013. Influence of implantation age on school-age language performance in pediatric cochlear implant users. *International Journal of Audiology* 52(4):219–229.

Tomblin, J. B., B. A. Barker, L. J. Spencer, X. Zhang, and B. J. Gantz. 2005. The effect of age at cochlear implant initial stimulation on expressive language growth in infants and toddlers. *Journal of Speech, Language, and Hearing Research* 48(4):853–867.

Walker, E. A., R. W. McCreery, M. Spratford, J. J. Oleson, J. Van Buren, R. Bentler, P. Roush, and M. P. Moeller. 2015. Trends and predictors of longitudinal hearing aid use for children who are hard of hearing. *Ear and Hearing* 36:38S–47S.

Waltzman, S. B., and W. H. Shapiro. 1999. Cochlear implants in children. *Trends in Amplification* 4(4):143–162.

2

Considerations for Evaluating Hearing Function

This chapter provides background information on the characteristics of hearing tests, presentation level, and test setup as well as defines various important terms related to the assessment of speech perception and discusses other considerations concerned with evaluating hearing function. It provides the background material necessary to understand Statement of Task items 1, 2, and 3c. Those issues also will be addressed more specifically in the chapters that follow. The chapter also provides a brief overview of the many types of speech recognition tests, which are covered in more detail in Chapter 4.

AUDITORY PROCESSING: DETECTION AND PERCEPTION

Audiologists assess at least two distinct factors with respect to auditory processing: detection and perception. Detection, also referred to as sensation, is a lower-order sensory process characterized by the perceptual recognition or awareness of an auditory stimulus. An audiogram represents detection-based processes in such a way that audiometric thresholds represent the lowest level at which an individual can reliably detect tonal stimuli across the frequency range most important for speech recognition. Perception is a higher-order sensory process that requires that the detected stimulus be transmitted to the central auditory system. As such, the assessment of speech recognition represents various aspects of perception so that a listener's score represents first the detection (awareness) of the stimulus, then the discrimination (speech versus non-speech), identification (particular talker), and, ultimately, comprehension of the speech stimulus (Erber, 1982).

Sentence recognition relies heavily on "top-down processing" (i.e., neurocognitive processes that access prior linguistic knowledge necessary for understanding semantic context, that use auditory working memory, and that are dependent on processing speed—all of which play critical roles in decoding a degraded auditory signal). Individuals with severe-to-profound sensorineural hearing loss—particularly those using cochlear implants—report that speech recognition is much more difficult in the presence of background noise (e.g., Donaldson et al., 2009). Despite these subjective reports of communication difficulty in noise that is characteristic of everyday listening environments, cochlear implant recipients achieve normal to near-normal detection of sounds in their environment with cochlear implant–aided audiograms in the range of 20 to 30 dB HL (decibel hearing level) from 250 through 6,000 Hz (e.g., Skinner et al., 1997, 1999). Focusing simply on detection as shown on the aided audiogram leads to over-estimating the auditory and communication potential of cochlear implant recipients, as cochlear implants do not amplify sounds to improve normal hearing; instead, they give a person a representation of sounds in the environment, which in turn helps with understanding speech (NIDCD, 2017). Consequently, the success in treating hearing loss through the use of cochlear implants is measured through functional measures of auditory processing relating to perception, namely assessments of speech recognition.

Hearing tests for those with cochlear implants are different from those used for people using acoustic hearing. The ideal test for those with cochlear implants would be reliable, highly sensitive to different conditions, and correlate well with speech perception abilities in the real world (Cullington and Aidi, 2017; Mackersie, 2002). Across-test correlation, or agreement, is also an important consideration in the choice of measures used for hearing assessment. Additional considerations for the U.S. Social Security Administration (SSA) include testing for success in the workplace and testing in children who may be uncooperative or who have experienced delays in developing language or speech skills.

Labeled cochlear implant criteria vary across manufacturers. The least restrictive labeled indications for conventional adult cochlear implant candidacy include moderate to profound sensorineural hearing loss in both ears and sentence recognition test scores ≤ 50 percent in the ear to be implanted and ≤ 60 percent in the best-aided condition (Cochlear Americas, 2020). The least restrictive labeled indications for children 2 to 17 years include severe to profound hearing loss in both ears and limited benefit from hearing aids, defined as word recognition scores ≤ 30 percent on the Multisyllabic Neighborhood Test (MLNT) or the Lexical Neighborhood Test (LNT) (Cochlear Americas, 2020).

HEARING TEST CHARACTERISTICS

Because hearing is a complex process that involves several levels of sensory processing, there are multiple considerations that an audiologist must take into account when preparing to evaluate hearing. Hearing tests can be categorized by the level of auditory skills required to complete a task (Tye-Murray et al., 2014). N. P. Erber first described the categories of auditory assessment from most basic to most complex in the 1982 manuscript *Auditory Training*; these categories are sound awareness, sound discrimination, sound identification, and comprehension (Erber, 1982). Sound awareness is the most basic level of auditory function and refers to the ability to detect the presence or absence of sound. Sound discrimination refers to the ability to discriminate between sounds and to recognize changes in sound over time. Sound identification is the ability of the listener to label or categorize a sound. Comprehension is the highest level of auditory skills and requires the listener to understand and interpret the sound. Functional assessment of hearing draws on tests of each of those auditory skill levels. Each higher level of auditory skill level is dependent on auditory skills lower in the hierarchy. Auditory–verbal communication with other people in occupational settings requires functional ability at all four levels.

The interdependence across levels of auditory skills has led to two approaches to functional hearing assessment related to occupational settings. One approach attempts to estimate the impact of environmental factors on individual auditory skills by testing lower-level auditory skills in realistic listening environments (Soli et al., 2018). That approach is useful for predicting functional hearing abilities at the group level, but it is less useful for predicting performance at the individual level or for specific work environments (Soli et al., 2018). The other approach directly assesses higher-level auditory skills such as identification or comprehension and may also attempt to recreate elements of a real-world listening environment (McGregor, 2003). That higher-level approach, however, can be limited by specificity. For example, if the assessment is of hearing on a radio or telephone, it cannot generalize to other occupational activities such as face-to-face communication or to auditory signals from equipment. Thus, functional hearing assessments often combine lower- and higher-level approaches to better reflect hearing abilities that are more general and tasks that are more specific to a particular occupation (NASEM, 2019).

SSA currently employs a combination of tests of varying auditory skills, including pure tone testing, speech detection via speech reception threshold, and speech recognition (namely unaided monosyllabic word recognition). However, for individuals with cochlear implants, a similar assessment cannot be completed because cochlear implant recipients hear through their implanted device transmitted via an externally worn sound processor.

Furthermore, as mentioned in the introduction, the characterization of aided detection on the audiogram for a cochlear implant recipient does not accurately reflect functional performance on measures of speech recognition, which are critical for effective communication. As such, SSA currently relies on a single, higher-level test—the Hearing in Noise Test (HINT) sentences (Nilsson et al., 1994)—that assesses speech recognition in a quiet background with sentences presented in the sound field[1] via a loudspeaker placed at 0° azimuth (i.e., directly in front of the listener) (SSA, 2010).

PRESENTATION LEVEL AND TEST SETUP

The standard unit of measurement used to express the level of a sound is the decibel (dB). However, a description of the sound level in dB alone is not sufficient to characterize the magnitude of a signal because that description is completely dependent on the reference level against which it was compared. Sound pressure level (SPL) is a common measure of sound level, with units in dB, that describes the displacement of air molecules with reference to 20 micropascals (20 μPa). Calculation of dB requires a reference. dB SPL is the reference that most people are familiar with, and it is in reference to the pressure of the measured displacement of air molecules relative to the surrounding or ambient air pressure, the latter of which is 20 μPa. dB SPL can be measured with a single measurement microphone. For dB SPL, the calculation is 20 log10(p/po), where p is the physical sound pressure of the signal measured in Pa, and po is 20 μPa (the reference sound pressure measurement in air—ambient air pressure). So, if the physical measurement is 20 μPa, then the calculated level in SPL = 0 dB SPL.

Due to the structural, mechanical, and resonant characteristics of the human auditory system, sound detection (sensitivity) is not equivalent in dB SPL across the frequency range of human hearing. Specifically, humans are most sensitive in the mid-frequency range from 2,000 to 6,000 Hz, with detection thresholds being much higher (i.e., poorer hearing) for sounds that are lower or higher in frequency than sounds in this middle ground. In an effort to provide a norm-referenced scale of hearing detection across the audiometric frequency range—typically 250 through 8,000 Hz—the dB HL scale was created. In this dB HL scale the zero reference level is defined in such a way that mean audiometric detection thresholds in dB SPL for individuals with normal hearing are set to be 0 dB HL across all frequencies.

The dB HL scale is used to express audiometric thresholds for pure tones and for spondees[2] used to determine speech reception thresholds and

---

[1] A defined space containing sound waves; in this context, the room that the listener is in.

[2] Spondees refer to compound words consisting of two independent words spoken with equal stress such as "airplane," "birthday," "popcorn," etc.

also to characterize the presentation level of monosyllables for unaided word recognition. In other words, the use of the dB HL scale is limited to diagnostic audiology practices. The dB HL scale is not used as the unit of measurement or calibration for speech recognition assessment in the sound field because such assessment should be accomplished at speech levels typically encountered in everyday communicative environments, which are measured and expressed in dB SPL.

In the mid-1970s, the U.S. Environmental Protection Agency funded a study to characterize speech and environmental sound levels encountered in everyday listening environments (Pearsons, 1977). That study found that average "normal" conversational speech at average conversational distances (~1 meter) was at 60 dB SPL and that higher speech levels representative of raised (65 dB SPL), loud (74 dB SPL), or shouted (84 dB SPL) voices could not be sustained for extended periods of time—particularly in the presence of background noise—given the vocal effort required of the talker (Olsen, 1998; Pearsons, 1977). Given that 60 dB SPL represents average conversational speech levels, best practices recommendations, as included in the Minimum Speech Test Battery (Auditory Potential, 2011) and pediatric Minimum Speech Test Battery (MSTB) (Uhler et al., 2017) manuals, specify the use of recorded speech stimuli presented at 60 dB SPL for the assessment of speech recognition performance for both pre- and post-implant assessment. While it is possible to characterize speech levels in the sound field using the dB HL scale, accounting for across-frequency audibility in the free field would transform 60 dB SPL to 40 dB HL. However, because sound field calibration uses a free-field microphone attached to a sound level meter and sound level meters are not equipped with a dB HL reference, presentation levels for speech recognition testing obtained in a sound field are characterized in dB SPL. As such, a presentation level recommendation referencing dB HL for sound field assessment is not possible and would therefore be inappropriate.

Calibration of Speech Stimuli in the Sound Field

When an acoustic signal is presented in the sound field, the sound can be characterized in the near field and in the far field relative to the listener. In the near field, large changes in SPL are associated with small changes in distance from the loudspeaker. To avoid rapid changes in SPL at the ear should the listener move, the listener in sound field testing is placed between the near- and far-field boundaries. To achieve that, the loudspeaker is placed at approximately 1 meter from the listener (Dirks et al., 1976) and should not be situated close to the walls of the test booth or other reflective surfaces.

Speech stimulus calibration for sound field testing focuses on output-based calibration. Output-based calibration in the audiology clinic is achieved by varying the audiometer dial setting, in dB HL, to achieve the desired presentation level in the sound field, in dB SPL, as measured with a sound level meter (SLM). The SLM with an attached free field microphone is generally placed on a stand and placed at the position of the listener's head when seated in a chair. This height is approximately 39 inches (86 cm) from the floor, which is also the recommended height of the loudspeaker (Auditory Potential, 2011). For sound field calibration, a calibration noise is required as the use of a calibration tone would result in standing waves in the free field. The calibration noise is normalized to the root mean square level of the accompanying speech stimuli. Thus, the clinician adjusts the audiometer dial in 1 dB increments to achieve a level of 60 dB SPL as shown on the SLM. The numerical reference on the audiometer dial setting (in dB HL) will likely not match the numerical level of the dB SPL reading. This mismatch between dB SPL and dB HL reading on the audiometer is expected and is related to the input level of the stimulus as saved to a compact disc or, if speech stimuli saved to an attached computer are being played, is related to the sound card specifications.

Most clinicians are familiar with the use of calibration tones, which are critical for input-based calibration completed for unaided speech audiometry, such as with spondees and monosyllables. However, it is not necessary to complete input-based calibration for sound field testing except to ensure that the input stimulus and audiometer sensitivity setting (EXT A or B)[3] are not resulting in the stimulus being clipped. That would be evident by a peaking response on the VU meter[4] of the audiometer. Note that if the input sensitivity for EXT A or B or the computer master volume is adjusted in any way after output calibration has been completed in the sound field, then the output-based calibration must be repeated. That is a quick and simple step to ensure that the audiometer's dial setting yields 60 dB SPL in the sound field.

Ideally, speech stimuli presented in the sound field should be calibrated every day prior to each sound field assessment of speech recognition; however, unless a clinic owns a SLM dedicated for sound field calibration, that is not a realistic expectation. The next best option would be daily calibration, because sound field assessment of speech recognition performance without prior calibration might result in an inaccurate description of a listener's auditory performance at the desired presentation level. Furthermore, without calibration the tester could potentially under- or over-estimate speech recognition for patients as the tester could be presenting at a much lower or higher presentation level than intended. That is particularly true if

---

[3] EXT A or B refers to the external input setting or the auxiliary input for the audiometer.

[4] VU meter refers to a volume unit meter, which is a device that displays a representation of the signal level in audio equipment.

a clinic is using digitized/computerized speech stimuli, as the master volume on the computer might be accidentally adjusted between assessments. For audiology clinics where daily access to a SLM is not possible, clinicians can access a variety of SLM applications from any smartphone. More important than the specific app itself is that the clinician tests the accuracy of the SLM app using the smartphone-integrated microphone against the calibrated SLM with a free-field microphone.

Speech Recognition in Quiet Versus Noise

Improvements in cochlear implant technology and the expansion of adult implant indications have produced increasing levels of speech recognition in quiet, to the point that unilateral cochlear implant recipients with post-lingual onset of deafness are routinely achieving 60 percent open-set[5] word recognition, on average (e.g., Buchman et al., 2020; Holden et al., 2013). That outcome is essentially double what was reported for adults with the first generation cochlear implant system (Skinner et al., 1994). Indeed, an increasingly higher proportion of adult and pediatric implant recipients demonstrate at or near ceiling-level performance for sentence recognition in quiet (Dunn et al., 2020; Gifford et al., 2018). Despite that great success, most cochlear implant recipients exhibit significant communication difficulty in the presence of background noise, with mean scores dropping by 30 to 40 percentage points at +5 dB signal-to-noise ratio (SNR)[6] as compared with scores in quiet (e.g., Dunn et al., 2020; Gifford et al., 2018). In everyday listening environments such as restaurants, train stations, and department stores, +5 dB is the most common SNR experienced, providing evidence for the ecologic validity of speech recognition in noise assessments (Pearsons et al., 1977; Smeds et al., 2015). For that reason, both the adult and pediatric MSTB[7] have recommended assessment of speech recognition

---

[5] Open set versus closed set: Closed-set tests are designed with a fixed number of possible responses such as are encountered in a multiple-choice exam or a speech recognition task for which the listener must pick the correct word from a fixed set of words provided to the listener. Open-set tasks are designed without limitations on the possible responses, such as essay questions on an exam or speech recognition tasks for which the listener must indicate their responses without any prompts.

[6] Although the term "signal-to-noise ratio (SNR)" is commonly used in audiology and hearing science to describe the level difference between the target signal (typically speech) and the background noise, it is actually a misnomer. For example, if the background noise level is 60 dB SPL and the target speech signal is 65 dB SPL, the SNR would be described as 5 dB. The term "ratio" is a misnomer because a mathematical ratio is a quotient, whereas, because decibels are defined in terms of logarithms, an SNR is actually a difference score (although it does correspond to a ratio).

[7] MSTB is the Minimum Speech Test Battery (Auditory Potential, 2011), designed to document word recognition in bilaterally hearing impaired cochlear implant individuals.

in noise using a +5 dB SNR to describe receptive communication abilities for patients in realistic listening scenarios (Auditory Potential, 2011; Uhler et al., 2017).

Hearing Configuration: Unilateral and Bilateral Cochlear Implants

A number of studies have compared bilateral and unilateral cochlear implant recipients using open-set sentence tests including the Bamford-Kowal-Bench Speech-in-Noise Test (BKB-SIN), the HINT, and the Maryland consonant–nucleus-consonant (CNC) word test (Dorman et al., 2011). The primary findings are briefly described below as well as in Table 2-1, which provides additional information.

Speech recognition performance significantly increased over the first 6 months of cochlear implant use for all conditions tested (ear cochlear implant alone and bilateral cochlear implant) (Buss et al., 2008; Koch et al., 2010; Litovsky et al., 2006).

On average, speech recognition in the bilateral cochlear implant condition was significantly higher than either cochlear implant alone for words (Buss et al., 2008; Koch et al., 2010; Litovsky et al., 2006), sentences (Buss et al., 2008; Koch et al., 2010; Litovsky et al., 2006), and sentences in noise (Buss et al., 2008; Koch et al., 2010; Litovsky et al., 2004, 2006).

Speech recognition performance for each cochlear implant alone (Eapen et al., 2009) and bilateral cochlear implant (Chang et al., 2010; Eapen et al., 2009) was stable over 4–6 years following cochlear implant activation.

Verification of Cochlear Implant Function

The American Academy of Audiology's Guidelines for the Audiologic Management of Adult Hearing Impairment specifies that verification of hearing aid function should be completed via probe microphone measurements in the ear canal to ensure that the prescribed gain and output are achieved using a validated prescriptive fitting formula (Valente et al., 2006). In fact, hearing aid audibility is typically measured via sound pressure level (SPL) in the ear canal at various input signal levels over the range typical of conversational speech, from casual (55 dB SPL) to average (60 dB SPL) and up to raised/loud speech (70 dB SPL) (Olsen, 1998; Pearsons et al., 1977). However, for cochlear implant verification, it is difficult to directly measure a physical output level because cochlear implants provide a transcutaneous transmission of the incoming stimulus to the implanted system using a radio frequency signal. That requires the use of behavioral responses to acoustic stimuli presented in the sound field as a measure of low-level audibility in cochlear implant users.

TABLE 2-1 Comparison of Open-Set Sentence and Monosyllabic Word Recognition in Adults with Simultaneous Bilateral Cochlear Implants

Outcome Measure	Scoring Method	Reference (Sample Size)	Results
HINT sentences in quiet	% correct	(1) Litovsky et al., 2006 (33) (2) Koch et al., 2010 (15)	(1) Performance improved from 1 to 6 months of cochlear implant use. (1 and 2) No significant difference between individual ear scores at any time point from pre-operation to 6 months post-operation; binaural summation at all time points (10 percentage points, on average); average bilateral HINT score reached 90 percent correct by 6 to 8 months. (2) Performance significantly improved from 6 to 8 months of cochlear use.
CNC words in quiet	% correct	(1) Litovsky et al., 2006 (33) (2) Koch et al., 2010 (15) (3) Buss et al., 2008 (26) (4) Eapen et al., 2009 (9) (5) Chang et al., 2010 (48)	(1–3) No significant difference between individual ear scores at any time point; binaural summation at all time points (10 percentage points, on average). (1–5) Average bilateral CNC score was 60 percent by 6–12 months of cochlear implant use. (4 and 5) Bilateral CNC scores were stable from 6 months up to 4–6 years.
BKB-SIN	SNR-50 (dB) S_0N_0	(1) Litovsky et al., 2006 (33) (2) Litovsky et al., 2009 (17)	(1 and 2) 2–3 dB bilateral benefit (binaural summation) over either unilateral cochlear implant alone. (1) Some listeners exhibited significant differences across ears, despite no interaural differences for speech in quiet.

NOTE: CNC = consonant–nucleus–consonant test; dB = decibel; HINT = Hearing in Noise Test; S_0N_0 = speech and noise both presented at 0° azimuth; SNR = signal-to-noise ratio.

Cochlear implant–aided sound field thresholds are critical for programming verification to ensure the audibility of low-level stimuli, such as soft speech. Skinner and colleagues first discussed the importance of sound field audiometric thresholds in the range of 20–30 dB HL for determining the minimum audibility available for implant recipients (Skinner et al., 1997, 1999), and there are now a number of published papers demonstrating that aided thresholds in the range of 20–25 dB HL are associated with significantly higher speech recognition outcomes for adult and pediatric cochlear implant recipients (e.g., Davidson et al., 2009; de Graaff et al., 2020; Holden et al., 2013, 2019). Thus, it is recommended that prior to assessing speech recognition abilities for cochlear implant recipients, aided sound field thresholds to warbled (frequency-modulated) pure tones are documented in the range of 20–30 dB HL from 250 through 6,000 Hz.

If aided thresholds are higher (i.e., poorer hearing) than the 20–30 dB range, the two most likely causes are implant processor microphone fidelity or suboptimal cochlear implant programming. For patients showing elevated aided thresholds, particularly in the high-frequency region, microphone fidelity may be suspect. It is recommended that a technician or audiologist listen to all implant processor microphones to check for static, low-level humming, or any evidence of compromised sound quality. Microphone issues often can be resolved via the replacement of microphone covers or filters on the implant sound processor. Less often, microphone issues will require processor repair or replacement. In cases where aided sound field thresholds are poor and microphone issues are ruled out, the most likely solution will be additional cochlear implant programming focusing first on lower stimulation levels (often called threshold or T levels). Increasing lower stimulation levels will generally result in better aided detection thresholds, although the exact levels at which T levels are set varies by each of the implant manufacturers. Note that each implanted ear should be verified independently to verify appropriate programming for each ear. Also, unilateral cochlear implant recipients who have some acoustic hearing in the non-implanted ear should have that ear occluded via foam plug or by a completely occluding earmold so that the implant ear is isolated for sound field testing. It is necessary to verify proper function of the cochlear implant(s) prior to assessing any speech reception in a sound field to ensure that the wearer's best performance is captured.

Aided Versus Unaided Speech Recognition Assessment

As mentioned above, audiologists routinely complete both unaided and aided speech recognition testing. Unaided speech recognition is most common in audiology practice as it involves threshold-based measures such as a speech reception threshold (SRT) and unaided word recognition testing at a suprathreshold level—typically in the range of 20 to 40 dB above SRT (Guthrie and Mackersie, 2009). Threshold and suprathreshold speech assessments should always include the use of recorded materials for standardized assessment across clinics and test administrators and to allow accurate tracking of performance over time. However, it has been reported that more than two-thirds of audiologists routinely use monitored live voice (MLV) for speech recognition assessments (Martin et al., 1998; Medwetsky et al., 1999). Roeser and Clark (2008) assessed word recognition obtained via MLV and recorded stimuli for 16 adult participants (32 ears) and found that word recognition scores for MLV and recorded stimuli were significantly different for 23 of the 32 ears (72 percent of the sample).

Furthermore, the difference between the MLV and recorded speech recognition scores was as high as 80 percentage points. In a similar study of 29 pediatric cochlear implant recipients aged 4 to 17 years, Uhler et al. (2016) assessed word and sentence recognition via MLV and recorded stimuli. They observed a 13 percentage point difference (range: 0 to 28 percentage points) between MLV and recorded stimulus presentation, which was found to be statistically significant.

There is a place for both unaided and aided assessments of suprathreshold speech recognition. As mentioned above, unaided assessments are typically conducted at levels 20–40 dB above the SRT, in dB HL. As an example, for a listener with a moderate to severe hearing loss exhibiting a 60 dB HL SRT, unaided word recognition would be tested in the range of 80–100 dB HL, corresponding to a range of approximately 100–120 dB SPL. Although unaided word recognition testing does not apply frequency-specific amplification to compensate for a listener's hearing loss, testing at such high presentation levels often results in better speech recognition scores than one would obtain in everyday listening scenarios where speech levels range from 55 to 70 dB SPL (Olsen, 1998; Pearsons, 1977). To gain a comprehensive profile of an individual's auditory skills in various communicative environments, unaided speech recognition should be paired with aided speech recognition—both in quiet and in noise—at an everyday conversational level, usually 60 dB SPL in quiet and 65 dB SPL in the presence of noise (Pearsons, 1977; Uhler et al., 2017).

INTRODUCTION TO SPEECH TESTS

Assessment of speech recognition taxes the central auditory system by requiring perception-based processing that involves discrimination, identification, and comprehension to various degrees (Erber, 1982). There are many available speech tests that are used to assess auditory function in individuals with cochlear implants. An overview of these tests can be found in Table 2-2. For additional information on each of the tests, please see Chapter 4.

Scoring Speech-in-Noise Tests

Clinical speech-in-noise tests are commonly scored using one of two methods. The most common scoring method for cochlear implant recipients is "percent correct based," reporting the percentage of words repeated correctly across a list of sentences presented at a fixed SNR, such as +5 dB SNR. In that particular example, the speech stimuli would be presented 5 dB higher than the background noise. The second most common scoring method for cochlear implant recipients is "threshold based," reporting the

TABLE 2-2 Commonly Used Speech Perception Tests

Speech Perception Test	Target Population	General Overview	Scoring	Reference
Word Tests				
WIN (Words in Noise)	Adults	Monosyllabic words presented at an adaptive level in fixed multi-talker babble	SNR-50	Wilson, 2003; Wilson and Burks, 2005
Digit Triplet	Adults	Digit triplets adaptively presented in fixed noise	Speech reception threshold	Smits et al., 2013
MLNT (Multisyllabic Lexical Neighborhood Test)	Children	Multisyllabic words presented at fixed level	Percent correct	Kirk et al., 1995
LNT (Lexical Neighborhood Test)	Children	Monosyllabic words presented at fixed level	Percent correct	Kirk et al., 1995
CNC (Consonant–Nucleus–Consonant)	Adult	Monosyllabic word lists presented at fixed level	Percent correct	Causey et al., 1984
NU6 (Northwestern University Test No. 6)	Adult	Monosyllabic word lists presented at fixed level	Percent correct	Tillman and Carhart, 1966
PBK (Phonetically Balanced Kindergarten)	Children	Monosyllabic word lists presented at a fixed level	Percent correct	Haskins, 1949
Sentence Tests				
HINT (Hearing in Noise Test)	Adults	Sentences presented at an adaptive level in fixed multi-talker babble	SNR loss/SNR-50	Nilsson et al., 1994

TABLE 2-2 Continued

Speech Perception Test	Target Population	General Overview	Scoring	Reference
HINT-C (Hearing in Noise Test-Children)	Children	Sentences presented at an adaptive level in fixed multi-talker babble	SNR loss/SNR-50	Nilsson et al., 1996
BKB-SIN (Bamford-Kowal-Bench Speech in Noise Test)	Adults and children	Sentences presented in four-talker babble with up to eight predetermined SNR levels	SNR loss/SNR-50	Etymōtic Research, 2005
QuickSIN (Quick Speech in Noise)	Adults	Sentences presented in multi-talker babble at six predetermined SNR levels	SNR loss/SNR-50	Killion et al., 2004
AzBio (Arizona Biomedical)	Adults	Sentences presented in 10-talker babble at a fixed SNR	Percent correct	Spahr et al., 2012
Pediatric AzBio	Children	Sentences presented in 10-talker babble at a fixed SNR	Percent correct	Spahr et al., 2014
CID Sentences (Central Institute for the Deaf)	Adults	Sentences presented at a fixed level, in quiet or noise	Percent correct	Silverman and Hirsh, 1955
CUNY Sentences (City University of New York)		Sentences presented at a fixed level, in quiet or noise	Percent correct	Boothroyd et al., 1985

NOTE: SNR = signal-to-noise ratio; SNR-50: "threshold-based" scoring reporting the SNR needed to obtain 50 percent correct recognition, measured in decibels.

SNR needed to obtain 50 percent correct recognition, measured in dB. In other words, during the test, the background noise (steady state noise or multi-talker babble) is increased to the point at which the listener can correctly identify 50 percent of the words or sentences, and the difference between the signal and noise is recorded as the listener's threshold in dB (e.g., Donaldson et al., 2009; Wilson et al., 2007).

The threshold-based method for scoring speech recognition in noise was originally employed using a psychophysical "staircase" procedure in which the level of the background noise is adaptively varied for each sentence based on the listener's prior response (Leek, 2001). For example, if a listener correctly repeats a sentence, the noise is increased for the following sentence. Conversely, if the patient cannot accurately repeat all words in a sentence for a given SNR, the noise is decreased for the following sentence. In the traditional adaptive staircase procedure, the SNR yielding 50 percent correct is calculated as the average SNR for the last 6 to 8 "reversal points" as it captures the SNR around which the listener achieves approximately 50 percent correct (e.g., Leek, 2001; Nilsson et al., 1994).

The adaptive staircase procedure for threshold-based scoring of speech recognition in noise is not clinically feasible because of time constraints and the need for specialized equipment and software. Thus, for clinical administration of threshold-based measures of speech recognition in noise, the 50 percent point is calculated using the Spearman-Karber equation (Finney, 1952), which can be done across various speech tests in noise, including the digit triplet test (Smits et al., 2004), the Words in Noise test (WIN; Wilson et al., 2007), the QuickSIN (Killion et al., 2004), and the BKB-SIN (Etymōtic Research, 2005). The Spearman-Karber equation (Finney, 1952) is 50 percent = i + ½(d) − (d)(# correct) / (w), where i = the initial presentation level (dB S/B[8]), d = the attenuation step size (decrement), and w = the number of items per decrement (Wilson et al., 2007).

Sentence Tests and Word Tests

SSA currently uses HINT sentences presented in a quiet background to assess hearing in individuals with cochlear implants at the *Listing of Impairments* (the Listings) level. The HINT corpus is a list of 25 everyday sentence lists spoken by a single male speaker.

The HINT is an adaptive speech recognition task (i.e., the level of each sentence is adjusted based on the response of the listener). The speech presentation level is decreased after each correct response, which raises the level of difficulty for the next sentence on the list. Conversely, the presentation level is increased after each incorrect response, which reduces the

---

[8] Signal-to-babble ratio.

difficulty for the following sentence. The level of the noise is held constant, thus adapting the presentation level of the sentences results in assessment at various SNRs.

The adaptive nature of the HINT ensures that the listener will approach a 50 percent correct response rate. Note that the HINT sentences can also be administered without noise in order to assess sentence recognition in quiet. In that case, a threshold for sentence recognition is obtained. If the test is administered in noise, adapting the SNR allows for the estimation of a SNR threshold for speech recognition in noise. As the SNR score decreases, the listening conditions become more difficult. For instance, if a hard-of-hearing listener is able to understand speech at an SNR of –3 dB in an omnidirectional hearing aid setting, then that individual may be able to understand speech at an SNR of –6 dB when the microphone setting has been changed to be directional. The change in microphone allows the listener to understand speech under more adverse conditions, thus improving his or her speech recognition ability in noise. However, everyday sentences inherently contain contextual cues for identification of individual words. Indeed, the HINT sentences contain five words per sentence, on average, and the language is consistent with a first-grade reading level, as evidenced by Flesch-Kincaid grade level assessment (Flesch, 1948; Kincaid et al., 1975).

An obvious concern with the use of speech tests is the extent to which context clues influence overall performance, which is dependent on the interaction between these context clues and a listener's knowledge of the language. Such an interaction might mean, for example, that subjects who are native speakers of the test language would yield norms that are inappropriate for nonnative speakers (NRC, 2005). The current Listing for hearing addresses this issue by noting,

> If you are not fluent in English, you should have word recognition testing using an appropriate word list for the language in which you are most fluent. The person conducting the test should be fluent in the language used for the test. If there is no appropriate word list or no person who is fluent in the language and qualified to perform the test, it may not be possible to measure your word recognition ability (2.00B4).

A second concern with the use of speech tests is the method of scoring sentence recognition performance, although most contemporary sentence tests assess accuracy based on the recognition of keywords. A third concern is whether the test has been standardized in quiet, noise, or both environmental conditions (NRC, 2005). As mentioned previously, the HINT sentence test was both developed and validated as a measure to be presented in an adaptive, staircase procedure in the presence of steady-state noise (Nilsson et al., 1994). Thus, the use of HINT sentences in a quiet background—or even in the presence of a fixed-SNR noise—is not consistent with the test's standardization and normative data. Furthermore, as discussed previously, the high level of specificity might not apply to the working environment of the individual taking the test.

Thus, sentence tests, including the HINT, the BKB-SIN, and the QuickSIN, all provide varying degrees of context cues to the listener (Wilson et al., 2007). By contrast, word tests using monosyllabic or bisyllabic words test a listener's ability to recognize discrete phonemes. These tests are typically conducted in quiet (Martin et al., 1998). Each test involves presenting full lists of the recorded materials (usually 50 words). Performance is quantified by a percentage correct score (NRC, 2005). Additionally, mono- and bisyllabic tests benefit from not being influenced by linguistic context or memory (Massa and Ruckenstein, 2014; McArdle et al., 2005). Those issues will be discussed further in Chapter 3.

REFERENCES

Auditory Potential. 2011. *Minimum Speech Test Battery for adult cochlear implant users.* http://www.auditorypotential.com/MSTBfiles/MSTBManual2011-06-20%20.pdf (accessed October 17, 2020).

Boothroyd, A. 1985. Evaluation of speech production of the hearing impaired: Some benefits of forced-choice testing. *Journal of Speech and Hearing Research* 28(2):185–196.

Buchman, C. A., R. H. Gifford, D. S. Haynes, T. Lenarz, G. O'Donoghue, O. Adunka, A. Biever, R. J. Briggs, M. L. Carlson, P. Dai, C. L. Driscoll, H. W. Francis, B. J. Gantz, R. K. Gurgel, M. R. Hansen, M. Holcomb, E. Karltorp, M. Kirtane, J. Larky, E. A. M. Mylanus, J. Thomas Roland, Jr., S. R. Saeed, H. Skarzynski, P. H. Skarzynski, M. Syms, H. Teagle, P. H. van de Heyning, C. Vincent, H. Wu, T. Yamasoba, and T. Zwolan. 2020. Unilateral cochlear implants for severe, profound, or moderate sloping to profound bilateral sensorineural hearing loss a systematic review and consensus statements. *JAMA Otolaryngology—Head and Neck Surgery* 146(10):942–953.

Buss, E., H. C. Pillsbury, C. A. Buchman, C. H. Pillsbury, M. S. Clark, D. S. Haynes, R. F. Labadie, S. Amberg, P. S. Roland, P. Kruger, M. A. Novak, J. A. Wirth, J. M. Black, R. Peters, J. Lake, P. A. Wackym, J. B. Firszt, B. S. Wilson, D. T. Lawson, R. Schatzer, P. S. C. D'Haese, and A. L. Barco. 2008. Multicenter U.S. bilateral MED-EL cochlear implantation study: Speech perception over the first year of use. *Ear and Hearing* 29(1):20–32.

Causey, G. D., L. J. Hood, C. L. Hermanson, and L. S. Bowling. 1984. The Maryland CNC test: Normative studies. *International Journal of Audiology* 23(6):552–568.

Chang, S. A., R. S. Tyler, C. C. Dunn, H. Ji, S. A. Witt, B. Gantz, and M. Hansen. 2010. Performance over time on adults with simultaneous bilateral cochlear implants. *Journal of the American Academy of Audiology* 21(1):35–43.

Cochlear Americas. 2020. *Nucleus cochlear implants: Physician's package insert.* https://www.accessdata.fda.gov/cdrh_docs/pdf/P970051S172C.pdf (accessed September 2, 2020).

Cullington, H. E., and T. Aidi. 2017. Is the digit triplet test an effective and acceptable way to assess speech recognition in adults using cochlear implants in a home environment? *Cochlear Implants International* 18(2):97–105.

Davidson, L. S., M. W. Skinner, B. A. Holstad, B. T. Fears, M. K. Richter, M. Matusofsky, C. Brenner, T. Holden, A. Birath, J. L. Kettel, and S. Scollie. 2009. The effect of instantaneous input dynamic range setting on the speech perception of children with the Nucleus 24 implant. *Ear and Hearing* 30(3):340–349.

de Graaff, F., B. I. Lissenberg-Witte, M. W. Kaandorp, P. Merkus, S. T. Goverts, S. E. Kramer, and C. Smits. 2020. Relationship between speech recognition in quiet and noise and fitting parameters, impedances and ECAP thresholds in adult cochlear implant users. *Ear and Hearing* 41(4):935–947.

Dirks, D. D., C. Kamm, and S. Gilman. 1976. Bone conduction thresholds for normal listeners in force and acceleration units. *Journal of Speech and Hearing Research* 19(1):181–186.

Donaldson, G. S., T. H. Chisolm, G. P. Blasco, L. J. Shinnick, K. J. Ketter, and J. C. Krause. 2009. BKB-SIN and ANL predict perceived communication ability in cochlear implant users. *Ear and Hearing* 30(4):401–410.

Dorman, M. F., W. A. Yost, B. S. Wilson, and R. H. Gifford. 2011. Speech perception and sound localization by adults with bilateral cochlear implants. *Seminars in Hearing* 32(1):73–89.

Dunn, C. C., J. Oleson, A. Parkinson, M. R. Hansen, and B. J. Gantz. 2020. Nucleus Hybrid S12: Multicenter clinical trial results. *Laryngoscope* 130(10):E548–E558.

Eapen, R. J., E. Buss, M. C. Adunka, H. C. Pillsbury, and C. A. Buchman. 2009. Hearing-in-noise benefits after bilateral simultaneous cochlear implantation continue to improve 4 years after implantation. *Otology and Neurotology* 30(2):153–159.

Erber, N. P. 1982. *Auditory training*. Washington, DC: Alexander Graham Bell Association for the Deaf.

Etymōtic Research. 2005. *BKB-SIN user's manual*. https://www.etymotic.com/downloads/dl/file/id/260/product/160/bkb_sintm_user_manual.pdf (accessed October 17, 2020).

Finney, D. J. 1952. *Statistical method in biological assay*. London, UK: C. Griffen.

Flesch, R. 1948. A new readability yardstick. *Journal of Applied Psychology* 32(3):221–233.

Gifford, R. H., L. Loiselle, S. Natale, S. W. Sheffield, L. W. Sunderhaus, M. S. Dietrich, and M. F. Dorman. 2018. Speech understanding in noise for adults with cochlear implants: Effects of hearing configuration, source location certainty, and head movement. *Journal of Speech, Language, and Hearing Research* 61(5):1306–1321.

Guthrie, L. A., and C. L. Mackersie. 2009. A comparison of presentation levels to maximize word recognition scores. *Journal of the American Academy of Audiology* 20(6):381–390.

Haskins, H. 1949. *A phonetically balanced test of speech discrimination for children*. Evanston, IL: Northwestern University.

Holden, L. K., C. Brenner, R. M. Reeder, and J. B. Firszt. 2013. Postlingual adult performance in noise with HiRes 120 and ClearVoice Low, Medium, and High. *Cochlear Implants International* 14(5):276–286.

Holden, L. K., J. B. Firszt, R. M. Reeder, N. Y. Dwyer, A. L. Stein, and L. M. Litvak. 2019. Evaluation of a new algorithm to optimize audibility in cochlear implant recipients. *Ear and Hearing* 40(4):990–1000.

Killion, M. C., P. A. Niquette, G. I. Gudmundsen, L. J. Revit, and S. Banerjee. 2004. Development of a Quick Speech-in-Noise Test for measuring signal-to-noise ratio loss in normal-hearing and hearing-impaired listeners. *Journal of the Acoustical Society of America* 116(4 I):2395–2405.

Kincaid, J. P., R. P. Fishburne, Jr., R. L. Rogers, and B. S. Chissom. 1975. *Derivation of new readability formulas (Automated Readability Index, Fog Count and Flesch Reading Ease Formula) for Navy enlisted personnel*. Research branch report 8-75. Millington, TN: Institute for Simulation and Training.

Kirk, K. I., D. B. Pisoni, and M. J. Osberger. 1995. Lexical effects on spoken word recognition by pediatric cochlear implant users. *Ear and Hearing* 16(5):470–481.

Koch, D. B., S. D. Soli, M. Downing, and M. J. Osberger. 2010. Simultaneous bilateral cochlear implantation: Prospective study in adults. *Cochlear Implants International* 11(2):84–99.

Leek, M. R. 2001. Adaptive procedures in psychophysical research. *Perception and Psychophysics* 63(8):1279–1292.

Litovsky, R., A. Parkinson, J. Arcaroli, and C. Sammeth. 2006. Simultaneous bilateral cochlear implantation in adults: A multicenter clinical study. *Ear and Hearing* 27(6):714–731.

Mackersie, C. L. 2002. Tests of speech perception abilities. *Current Opinion in Otolaryngology and Head and Neck Surgery* 10(5):392–397.

Martin, F. N., C. A. Champlin, and J. A. Chambers. 1998. Seventh survey of audiometric practices in the United States. *Journal of the American Academy of Audiology* 9(2):95–104.

Massa, S. T., and M. J. Ruckenstein. 2014. Comparing the performance plateau in adult cochlear implant patients using HINT and AzBio. *Otology and Neurotology* 35(4):598–604.

McArdle, R. A., R. H. Wilson, and C. A. Burks. 2005. Speech recognition in multitalker babble using digits, words, and sentences. *Journal of the American Academy of Audiology* 16(9):726–739.

McGregor, A. 2003. Fitness standards in airline staff. *Occupational Medicine* 53(1):5–9.

Medwetsky, L., D. Sanderson, and D. Young. 1999. A national survey of audiology clinical practices. *The Hearing Review* 11:24–32.

NASEM (National Academies of Sciences, Engineering, and Medicine). 2019. *Functional assessment for adults with disabilities.* Washington, DC: The National Academies Press.

NIDCD (National Institute on Deafness and Other Communication Disorders). 2017 (March 6). *Cochlear implants.* https://www.nidcd.nih.gov/health/cochlear-implants (accessed August 19, 2020).

Nilsson, M., S. D. Soli, and J. A. Sullivan. 1994. Development of the Hearing in Noise Test for the measurement of speech reception thresholds in quiet and in noise. *Journal of the Acoustical Society of America* 95(2):1085–1099.

Nilsson, M. J., S. D. Soli, and D. J. Gelnett. 1996. *Development of the Hearing in Noise Test for Children (HINT-C).* Los Angeles, CA: House Ear Institute.

NRC (National Research Council). 2005. *Hearing loss: Determining eligibility for Social Security benefits.* Washington, DC: The National Academies Press.

Olsen, W. O. 1998. Average speech levels and spectra in various speaking/listening conditions: A summary of the Pearson, Bennett, & Fidell (1977) report. *American Journal of Audiology* 7(2):21–25.

Pearsons, K. S. 1977. Effect of tone/noise combination on speech intelligibility. *Journal of the Acoustical Society of America* 61(3):884–886.

Roeser, R. J., and J. L. Clark. 2008. Live voice speech recognition audiometry: Stop the madness! *Audiology Today* 20(1):32–33.

Silverman, S. R., and I. J. Hirsh. 1955. CX problems related to the use of speech in clinical audiometry. *Annals of Otology, Rhinology and Laryngology* 64(4):1234–1244.

Skinner, M. W., G. M. Clark, L. A. Whitford, P. M. Seligman, J. S. Staller, D. B. Shipp, J. K. Shallop, C. Everingham, C. M. Menapace, P. L. Arndt, T. Antogenelli, J. A. Brimacombe, S. Pijl, P. Daniels, C. R. George, H. J. McDermott, and A. L. Beiter. 1994. Evaluation of a new spectral peak coding strategy for the Nucleus 22-channel cochlear implant system. *American Journal of Otology* 15(Suppl 2):15–27.

Skinner, M. W., L. K. Holden, and T. A. Holden. 1997. Parameter selection to optimize speech recognition with the nucleus implant. *Otolaryngology—Head and Neck Surgery* 117(3 I):188–195.

Skinner, M. W., L. K. Holden, T. A. Holden, and M. E. Demorest. 1999. Comparison of two methods for selecting minimum stimulation levels used in programming the Nucleus 22 cochlear implant. *Journal of Speech, Language, and Hearing Research* 42(4):814–828.

Smeds, K., F. Wolters, and M. Rung. 2015. Estimation of signal-to-noise ratios in realistic sound scenarios. *Journal of the American Academy of Audiology* 26(2):183–196.

Smits, C., T. S. Kapteyn, and T. Houtgast. 2004. Development and validation of an automatic speech-in-noise screening test by telephone. *International Journal of Audiology* 43(1):15–28.

Smits, C., S. Theo Goverts, and J. M. Festen. 2013. The Digits-in-Noise Test: Assessing auditory speech recognition abilities in noise. *Journal of the Acoustical Society of America* 133(3):1693–1706.

Soli, S. D., C. Giguère, C. Laroche, V. Vaillancourt, W. A. Dreschler, K. S. Rhebergen, K. Harkins, M. Ruckstuhl, P. Ramulu, and L. S. Meyers. 2018. Evidence-based occupational hearing screening I: Modeling the effects of real-world noise environments on the likelihood of effective speech communication. *Ear and Hearing* 39(3):436–448.

Spahr, A. J., M. F. Dorman, L. M. Litvak, S. Van Wie, R. H. Gifford, P. C. Loizou, L. M. Loiselle, T. Oakes, and S. Cook. 2012. Development and validation of the AzBio sentence lists. *Ear and Hearing* 33(1):112–117.

Spahr, A. J., M. F. Dorman, L. M. Litvak, S. J. Cook, L. M. Loiselle, M. D. DeJong, A. Hedley-Williams, L. S. Sunderhaus, C. A. Hayes, and R. H. Gifford. 2014. Development and validation of the Pediatric AzBio sentence lists. *Ear and Hearing* 35(4):418–422.

SSA (U.S. Social Security Administration). 2010. Listing of Impairments—Adult listings (part A). In *The blue book*. Washington, DC: U.S. Social Security Administration.

Tillman, T. W., and R. Carhart. 1966. *An expanded test for speech discrimination utilizing CNC monosyllabic words: Northwestern University Auditory Test no. 6*. Technical report SAM-TR-66-55. Brooks Air Force Base, Texas: USAF School of Aerospace Medicine. https://pdfs.semanticscholar.org/008e/54f6708d34231a350af7e7b585b53a8c048c.pdf (accessed January 15, 2021).

Tye-Murray, N., S. Hale, B. Spehar, J. Myerson, and M. S. Sommers. 2014. Lipreading in school-age children: The roles of age, hearing status, and cognitive ability. *Journal of Speech, Language, and Hearing Research* 57(2):556–565.

Uhler, K., A. Biever, and R. H. Gifford. 2016. Method of speech stimulus presentation impacts pediatric speech recognition monitored live voice versus recorded speech. *Otology and Neurotology* 37(2):e70–e74.

Uhler, K., A. Warner-Czyz, and R. Gifford. 2017. Pediatric Minimum Speech Test Battery. *Journal of the American Academy of Audiology* 28(3):232–247.

Valente, M., D. Benson, T. Chisolm, D. Citron, D. Hampton, A. Loavenbruck, T. Ricketts, H. Solodar, and R. Sweetow. 2007. Guidelines for the Audiologic Management of Adult Hearing Impairment Task Force members. https://audiology-web.s3.amazonaws.com/migrated/haguidelines.pdf_53994876e92e42.70908344.pdf (accessed January 16, 2021).

Wilson, R. H. 2003. Development of a speech-in-multitalker-babble paradigm to assess word-recognition performance. *Journal of the American Academy of Audiology* 14(9):453–470.

Wilson, R. H., and C. A. Burks. 2005. Use of 35 words for evaluation of hearing loss in signal-to-babble ratio: A clinic protocol. *Journal of Rehabilitation Research and Development* 42(6):839–851.

Wilson, R. H., R. A. McArdle, and S. L. Smith. 2007. An evaluation of the BKB-SIN, HINT, QuickSIN, and WIN materials on listeners with normal hearing and listeners with hearing loss. *Journal of Speech, Language, and Hearing Research* 50(4):844–856.

3

Characteristics and Limitations of the Hearing in Noise Test

This chapter responds to the first item in the Statement of Task:

> [T]o identify and describe the salient test characteristics of the Hearing in Noise Test (HINT), which is currently used to determine the functional hearing ability in adults or children with hearing loss treated with cochlear implantation, and provide recommendations as to how to generalize those characteristics into criteria that can be applied to other validated hearing tests for persons with cochlear implants.

Although the chapter provides a description of the salient characteristics of the HINT, the committee believes that recommending how to generalize those characteristics to other validated tests is likely not the most useful question. As will be discussed, the HINT is no longer the most up-to-date or the most useful test for individuals with cochlear implants. This chapter and subsequent chapters will explain the committee's thinking and provide recommendations for useful criteria that can be applied to validated hearing tests for persons with cochlear implants.

BACKGROUND

The HINT was originally chosen by the U.S. Social Security Administration (SSA) because it was a widely available test. The SSA *Listing of Impairments* (the Listings) for hearing loss with cochlear implants in adults states:

a. If you have a cochlear implant, we will consider you to be disabled until 1 year after initial implantation.
b. After that period, we need word recognition testing performed with any version of the Hearing in Noise Test (HINT) to determine whether your impairment meets 2.11B. This testing must be conducted in quiet in a sound field. Your implant must be functioning properly and adjusted to your normal settings. The sentences should be presented at 60 dB HL (decibel hearing level) and without any visual cues (SSA, 2020).

At the time when that guidance was drafted, speech perception in noise for people with cochlear implants was still very poor, which resulted in the HINT sentences being administered in quiet. However, as cochlear implant technology continued to improve, it no longer made sense to administer the HINT in a quiet sound field, and audiologists today believe a more difficult test is needed to minimize ceiling effects.

Because the U.S. Food and Drug Administration (FDA) approved the use of cochlear implants for hearing loss in adults in 1984, the technology and the surgical techniques involved in its installation have improved considerably and have resulted in ever-improving outcomes for individuals with hearing loss. That has resulted in a continued need for updated materials and assessment criteria to match the improvements in cochlear implant devices.

Historically, the Central Institute for the Deaf (CID) sentence lists were used in cochlear implant research and candidacy. However, as the surgical techniques, technologic processing and components of cochlear implants, and audiologic rehabilitation regiments improved, so did cochlear implant outcomes. With that improvement, the relatively easy CID sentences fell out of favor due to ceiling effects exhibited in tests of cochlear implant recipients. In the 1990s the HINT sentences became the favored assessment for cochlear implantation. The HINT was developed by Nilsson et al. (1994) in response to the need for a broader assessment of speech ability and to address the floor and ceiling effects of the speech assessments that were being used in practice at that time (Nilsson et al., 1994).

DEVELOPMENT OF THE HEARING IN NOISE TEST

As noted in previous chapters, the HINT (Nilsson et al., 1994) is an adaptive speech-in-noise test that is composed of 250 sentences divided into 25 lists. The test is adaptive in that the signal-to-noise ratio (SNR) (see Chapter 2) is to be adjusted based on the performance of the participant. The HINT was designed and validated to fix the noise level and adjust the speech level adaptively based on the listener's responses. This means that for each sentence correctly repeated, the following sentence is presented at a lower volume, and for each sentence incorrectly repeated, the following sentence is presented at a higher volume. That adaptive tracking often referred to as a one-down, one-up tracking paradigm with the intention of converging on the SNR required for a score of 50 percent correct. The intended purpose of the adaptive style was to protect against ceiling effects such as those experienced by the relatively easier CID sentence lists at the time. Now, with the ongoing improvements in cochlear implants, the HINT is itself subject to the ceiling effects.

The HINT sentences are based on the Bamford-Kowal-Bench (BKB) sentences. The authors revised the 336 BKB sentences to remove British English idioms for an American English audience while maintaining the sentence length. They had native speakers of American English rate the naturalness of the sentences. The resulting sentences were recorded by a male speaker, and mean-squared amplitudes were calculated for each sentence waveform. All waveforms were rescaled to 67 dB to equate the initial presentation levels. In addition, the average long-term spectrum (i.e., average spectrum of all voiced sounds over the period of time of the presented sentence) were equated and used as a benchmark to generate a spectrally-matched (i.e., speech-shaped) noise masker. That form of masking is based on energy masking rather than on informational masking such as a multi-talker babble that contains other random speech. Some studies report speech-shaped masking as being more effective (i.e., the sentences are more difficult to understand). This association may be different in native English speakers than in those who speak English as a second language (Hall et al., 2002; Jin and Liu, 2012). Finally, sentence intelligibility was assessed based on phonemic content and word familiarity. To compensate for intelligibility and equate the difficulty across sentences, the authors increased the mean-squared level of the sentence waveform for sentences with below-average intelligibility (i.e., reduced the presented SNR to increase difficulty).

The modified 250 sentences chosen from the initial 336 BKB sentences were divided into 25 lists of 10 sentences that are matched for phonemic distribution. To assess inter-list reliability in quiet and fixed-noise, authors recruited 18 normal-hearing native English speakers who were presented lists of sentences in randomized order in quiet and noise conditions. Based on repeated measures within subjects, the authors reported a 95% confidence interval for 10-sentence lists estimated at ± 2.41 dB in noise and ± 2.98 dB in quiet. Average thresholds for the HINT were 23.91 dB in quiet and 69.08 dB in fixed noise (72 dB SPL [sound pressure level]). The authors further reported that a threshold measurement with a single list took less than 2 minutes during their study (Nilsson et al., 1994).

ADMINISTRATION OF THE HEARING IN NOISE TEST

For HINT administration in the aided condition, the test is designed to be administered with the participant sitting 1 meter from a loudspeaker that is placed directly in front of the individual (i.e., 0 degrees). The target speech stimuli are presented from the speaker at 0 degrees. The background noise was originally designed to be a steady-state, speech-shaped noise and was presented from the same loudspeaker so that the speech and noise were co-located. However, the HINT is also often presented with spatially separated speech and noise so that the noise originates from an angle of 90 or 270 degrees from the direction of the speech (e.g., Vermiglio, 2008; Vermiglio et al., 2020). Speech understanding in conditions with spatially separated speech and noise is less difficult than when speech and noise are coming from the same place because the listener can benefit from spatial release from masking (SRM). SRM is a phenomenon arising from both head shadow and an across-ear comparison of binaural cues—interaural level differences and interaural time differences—although there are additional cues that may play a role, including spatial attention and better-ear listening (Goupell et al., 2016).

For HINT administration in the unaided condition, the speech and noise stimuli are presented via supra aural headphones or insert earphones (Nilsson et al., 1994). Stimulus presentation can be unilateral or bilateral. In cases of unilateral HINT administration, the non-test ear may require masking so that individual ear performance is quantified. In addition to the standard materials and methods used in the development and validation of the HINT, several studies have administered the adaptive HINT via an eight-loudspeaker circumferential array with speech presented from 0 degrees and uncorrelated noise presented from all eight loudspeakers (e.g., Compton-Conley et al., 2004; Valente et al., 2006). In this scenario, speech and noise are both co-located (from the 0-degree loudspeaker) and spatially separated (for the noise from all of the other loudspeakers), presenting a much more difficult listening environment, given the diffuse nature of the noise. The eight-loudspeaker system is generally used in research laboratories and is not typically incorporated into clinical audiology protocols.

SALIENT CHARACTERISTICS OF THE HEARING IN NOISE TEST

The committee's Statement of Task directs it to detail the salient characteristics of the HINT. As designed, the HINT has the following characteristics (also see Table 3-1):

TABLE 3-1 Salient Characteristics of the Hearing in Noise Test (HINT)

Characteristic	Description
Sentences	The HINT is composed of 250 sentences that are divided into 25 lists
Adaptive assessment	The original design of the assessment uses an adaptive model to adjust the speech level to prevent ceiling effects[a]
Intelligibility of materials	Phonemic content and word familiarity based on American English are balanced across 25 lists of 10 sentences
Accessibility across multiple languages	Translated into at least 11 languages[b]
Speech-spectrum noise	Noise is spectrally matched to the amplitude and frequency response of the recorded sentences
Recorded speech by singular speaker	The HINT materials were recorded by a singular male speaker
Co-located speech and noise signals	Assessment designed presentation from a singular sound source (i.e., speech and noise come from the same speaker)
Quick assessment tool	Each sentence list from the HINT takes approximately 2 minutes to complete
Material access	At this time the HINT is difficult to obtain outside of large academic medical centers

[a] The intended use may not be consistent with actual use due to fixed-presentation recommendations from the Minimum Speech Test Battery in 1996.
[b] The clinician presenting the materials must be fluent in the language of administration.

- Uses sentences
- Adaptive assessment
- Intelligible materials
- Translated into multiple languages
- Speech-spectrum noise
- Recorded male speaker
- Designed for co-located speech from the same azimuth
- Relatively quick assessment
- Difficult to obtain

However, just as improvements in cochlear implant technology and surgical techniques warranted a change from CID to HINT sentences, recent improvements in these areas may warrant SSA re-evaluating its current use of the HINT.

THE HEARING IN NOISE TEST AS A TEST FOR INDIVIDUALS WITH COCHLEAR IMPLANTS

After its inception, the HINT became a widely used speech assessment tool. It has been used to assess communication disabilities among adults with hearing loss (Nilson et al., 1994) and in occupational assessments for hearing-critical jobs (Giguère et al., 2008; Soli et al., 2018a,b). A version has been adapted and validated for children (HINT-C) (Nilsson et al., 1996). It has been translated and validated in multiple languages.[1] Of note (and discussed in Chapter 2), the administrator of the HINT must be fluent in the language of the assessment. Additionally, one of its common uses has been as a tool for cochlear implant candidacy and outcomes assessment.

In 1996, stakeholders from otolaryngology, audiology, hearing science, and cochlear implant manufacturers recommended a Minimum Speech Test Battery (MSTB) for cochlear implant candidacy and for assessment of post-operative performance. At that meeting, both the consonant–nucleus–consonant (CNC) word test (Peterson and Lehiste, 1962) and the HINT (Nilsson et al., 1994) were recommended to assess patient performance prior to and following cochlear implantation. In breaking with the intended adaptive presentation format of the HINT, the committee recommended that two 10-sentence HINT lists be presented in quiet (65 A-weighted dB [dB A]) and at fixed-level noise with +10, +5, or 0 dB SNR (Gifford and Revit, 2010; Nilsson et al., 1996).

In 2001 a committee from the American Academy of Otolaryngology—Head and Neck Surgery updated the MSTB and recommended the HINT in its intended administration as an adaptive speech in noise test. However, that recommendation of the adaptive HINT was only intended for post-operative evaluation to avoid ceiling effects, while the HINT sentences in quiet at 70 dB SPL were recommended for preoperative evaluation (Gifford and Revit, 2010; Luxford, 2001). In 2011 the MSTB was revisited by the three manufacturers of cochlear implants in the United States, which resulted in the HINT sentences being dropped in favor of the more difficult, multi-talker Arizona Biomedical (AzBio) sentences (Spahr et al., 2012). The AzBio sentences include 660 sentences recorded from two female and two male speakers.

In the United States manufacturers have historically used the HINT sentences in quiet in the assessment of cochlear implant safety and effectiveness data for FDA. The HINT in quiet is a staple of candidacy indication from FDA-approved insert labeling for devices. Manufacturers used

---

[1] For example, Arabic (Essawy et al., 2019), Bulgarian (Lolov et al., 2008), Cantonese (Wong and Soli, 2005), French (Vaillancourt et al., 2005), Japanese (Shiroma et al., 2008), Korean (Moon et al., 2008), Malay (Quar et al., 2008), Mandarin (Fu et al., 2011; Wong et al., 2007), Norwegian (Myhrum and Moen, 2008), Portuguese (Bevilacqua et al., 2015), Spanish (Weiss and Dempsey, 2008), and Turkish (Cekic and Sennaroglu, 2008).

slightly different criteria with percent correct criteria, aided conditions, and presentation levels all varying across manufacturers (Gifford and Revit, 2010). Notably, the current Medicare criteria for cochlear implantation do not specify an assessment measure or presentation level, but rather provide general criteria of up to 40 percent correct in best-aided listening condition with tape-recorded open-set sentences (CMS, 2020; Gifford and Revit, 2010).

SSA requires audiometric testing for individuals with a cochlear implant. It considers a person with hearing loss disabled until age 5, or for 1 year after initial cochlear implantation, whichever is later. After that period SSA requires speech recognition testing performed with any version of the HINT to determine whether the person's impairment meets requirements for disability (SSA Listing 2.11B and 102.11B). The testing must be conducted in quiet in a sound field. The individual's implant must be functioning properly and adjusted to the person's normal settings. SSA requirements state that the sentences should be presented at 60 dB HL (Hearing Level) and without any visual cues (SSA Listing 102.00B3b). The current SSA use of the HINT dates back to 2008.[2]

LIMITATIONS OF THE HEARING IN NOISE TEST

Despite its common inclusion in candidacy and outcomes criteria for cochlear implant recipients, recent work has demonstrated that the HINT is limited by its administration, ceiling effects when presented in quiet or fixed SNRs, ecologic validity, and availability. While using the HINT as intended as an adaptive assessment may avoid ceiling effects, the test is commonly used in quiet or in fixed SNRs, as suggested in the previous MSTB documents (Luxford et al., 2001; Nilsson et al., 1996). This administration deviates from the adaptive presentation and results in ceiling effects that prevent appropriate performance monitoring over time (Gifford and Revit, 2010). In a study of 206 adults with hearing loss (156 cochlear implant recipients, 50 hearing aid users), Gifford et al. (2008) assessed performance on monosyllabic word (CNC) and sentence materials (e.g., the HINT, AzBio, BKB-SIN). The study found that 28 percent of the subjects achieved a maximum 100 percent correct score on the HINT when it was presented in quiet. Furthermore, of all the materials presented in quiet in the study, the HINT exhibited the highest percentage of ceiling effects (Gifford et al., 2008). Others have reported similar findings on ceiling effects. For example, a study of 78 adult cochlear implant users found that the HINT suffered from ceiling effects when presented in quiet at 70 and 60 dB SPL (although not when presented at 50 dB SPL or with background noise). In

---

[2] 73 FR 47103.

a retrospective chart review of adult cochlear implant outcomes, Massa and Ruckenstein (2014) also reported that the HINT Sentences test was more likely to suffer from ceiling effects than AzBio sentences.

As described above, the HINT was developed to keep the noise level fixed and adapt to the presentation level of speech. However, keeping the presentation level of speech constant may be a more relevant approach as talkers will be unable to adjust the level of their voice beyond 2–5 dB SNR in the presence of high-level background noise (e.g., Pearsons, 1977; Smeds et al., 2015). Moreover, the current scoring of the adaptive rule requires that the listener correctly repeat the entire sentence (Nilsson et al., 1994). While this has remained the primary adaptive protocol used for HINT administration, Chan et al. (2008) demonstrated the feasibility of using different adaptive rules tracking different points on the psychometric function allowing for 1–3 errors per sentence. The different methods were intended for use with individuals scoring at or near 50 percent in quiet, allowing the administration of the adaptive HINT across a broader range of listeners (Chan et al., 2008). While that remains a feasible method for adaptive HINT administration, the measure still offers limited ecologic validity, given the use of a single male talker, well-articulated speech, and a steady-state background noise. In addition to those issues, most clinics lack the tools necessary to quickly administer and score an adaptive measure within the confines of a clinical audiometric test suite.

In addition to ceiling effects, the lack of availability of the HINT materials has created problems. In historical context, with the conceptualization of the first MSTB in 1996, cochlear implant surgery was performed only at select major medical centers in the United States. Those centers were able to obtain the necessary test materials and had the appropriate equipment set up (i.e., speaker arrays) to perform speech performance assessments. However, due to its exclusion from the most recent MSTB and the fact that it is no longer available for purchase, the HINT is difficult for clinics across the United States to obtain.

REFERENCES

Bevilacqua, M. C., M. R. Banhara, E. A. Da Costa, A. B. Vignoly, and K. F. Alvarenga. 2008. The Brazilian Portuguese Hearing in Noise Test. *International Journal of Audiology* 47(6):364–365.

Cekic, S., and G. Sennaroglu. 2008. The Turkish Hearing in Noise Test. *International Journal of Audiology* 47(6):366–368.

Chan, A. S., M. C. Cheung, S. L. Sze, W. W. Leung, and R. W. Y. Cheung. 2008. Measuring vocabulary by free expression and recognition tasks: Implications for assessing children, adolescents, and young adults. *Journal of Clinical and Experimental Neuropsychology* 30(8):892–902.

CMS (Centers for Medicare & Medicaid Services). 2020. *Cochlear implantation.* https://www.cms.gov/Medicare/Coverage/Coverage-with-Evidence-Development/Cochlear-Implantation (accessed December 17, 2020).

Compton-Conley, C. L., A. C. Neuman, M. C. Killion, and H. Levitt. 2004. Performance of directional microphones for hearing aids: Real-world versus simulation. *Journal of the American Academy of Audiology* 15(6):440–455.

Essawy, W., E. Kolkaila, I. Kabbash, and A. Emara. 2019. Development and standardization of new hearing in noise test in Arabic language. *International Journal of Otorhinolaryngology and Head and Neck Surgery* 5:1501.

Fu, Q. J., M. Zhu, and X. Wang. 2011. Development and validation of the Mandarin speech perception test. *Journal of the Acoustical Society of America* 129(6):EL267–EL273.

Gifford, R. H., and L. J. Revit. 2010. Speech perception for adult cochlear implant recipients in a realistic background noise: Effectiveness of preprocessing strategies and external options for improving speech recognition in noise. *Journal of the American Academy of Audiology* 21(7):441–451.

Gifford, R. H., J. K. Shallop, and A. M. Peterson. 2008. Speech recognition materials and ceiling effects: Considerations for cochlear implant programs. *Audiology and Neurotology* 13(3):193–205.

Giguère, C., C. Laroche, S. D. Soli, and V. Vaillancourt. 2008. Functionally-based screening criteria for hearing-critical jobs based on the Hearing in Noise Test. *International Journal of Audiology* 47(6):319–328.

Goupell, M. J., A. Kan, and R. Y. Litovsky. 2016. Spatial attention in bilateral cochlear-implant users. *Journal of the Acoustical Society of America* 140(3):1652–1662.

Hall, J. W., III, J. H. Grose, E. Buss, and M. B. Dev. 2002. Spondee recognition in a two-talker masker and a speech-shaped noise masker in adults and children. *Ear and Hearing* 23(2):159–165.

Jin, S. H., and C. Liu. 2012. English sentence recognition in speech-shaped noise and multi-talker babble for English-, Chinese-, and Korean-native listeners. *Journal of the Acoustical Society of America* 132(5):EL391–EL397.

Lolov, S. R., A. M. Raynov, I. B. Boteva, and G. E. Edrev. 2008. The Bulgarian hearing in noise test. *International Journal of Audiology* 47(6):371–372.

Luxford, W. M. 2001. Minimum Speech Test Battery for postlingually deafened adult cochlear implant patients. *Otolaryngology—Head and Neck Surgery* 124(2):125–126.

Massa, S. T., and M. J. Ruckenstein. 2014. Comparing the performance plateau in adult cochlear implant patients using HINT and AzBio. *Otology and Neurotology* 35(4):598–604.

Moon, S. K., S. Hee Kim, H. Ah Mun, H. Kyung Jung, J. H. Lee, Y. H. Choung, and K. Park. 2008. The Korean Hearing in Noise Test. *International Journal of Audiology* 47(6):375–376.

Myhrum, M., and I. Moen. 2008. The Norwegian Hearing in Noise Test. *International Journal of Audiology* 47(6):377–378.

Nilsson, M., S. D. Soli, and J. A. Sullivan. 1994. Development of the Hearing in Noise Test for the measurement of speech reception thresholds in quiet and in noise. *Journal of the Acoustical Society of America* 95(2):1085–1099.

Nilsson, M. J., S. D. Soli, and D. J. Gelnett. 1996. *Development of the Hearing in Noise Test for Children (HINT-C).* Los Angeles, CA: House Ear Institute.

Pearsons, K. S. 1977. Effect of tone/noise combination on speech intelligibility. *Journal of the Acoustical Society of America* 61(3):884–886.

Peterson, G. E., and I. Lehiste. 1962. Revised CNC lists for auditory tests. *Journal of Speech and Hearing Disorders* 27:62–70.

Quar, K. T., Z. S. Mukari, A. A. N. Wahab, A. R. Razak, M. Omar, and N. Maamor. 2008. The Malay Hearing in Noise Test. *International Journal of Audiology* 47(6):379–380.

Shiroma, M., T. Iwaki, T. Kubo, and S. Soli. 2008. The Japanese hearing in noise test. *International Journal of Audiology* 47(6):381–382.

Smeds, K., F. Wolters, and M. Rung. 2015. Estimation of signal-to-noise ratios in realistic sound scenarios. *Journal of the American Academy of Audiology* 26(2):183–196.

Soli, S. D., C. Giguère, C. Laroche, V. Vaillancourt, W. A. Dreschler, K. S. Rhebergen, K. Harkins, M. Ruckstuhl, P. Ramulu, and L. S. Meyers. 2018a. Evidence-based occupational hearing screening I: Modeling the effects of real-world noise environments on the likelihood of effective speech communication. *Ear and Hearing* 39(3):436–448.

Soli, S. D., A. Amano-Kusumoto, O. Clavier, J. Wilbur, K. Casto, D. Freed, C. Laroche, V. Vaillancourt, C. Giguère, W. A. Dreschler, and K. S. Rhebergen. 2018b. Evidence-based occupational hearing screening II: Validation of a screening methodology using measures of functional hearing ability. *International Journal of Audiology* 57(5):323–334.

Spahr, A. J., M. F. Dorman, L. M. Litvak, S. Van Wie, R. H. Gifford, P. C. Loizou, L. M. Loiselle, T. Oakes, and S. Cook. 2012. Development and validation of the AzBio sentence lists. *Ear and Hearing* 33(1):112–117.

SSA (U.S. Social Security Administration). 2020. Disability evaluation under Social Security 2.00: Special senses and speech—Adult. In *The blue book*. Washington, DC: U.S. Social Security Administration.

Vaillancourt, V., C. Laroche, C. Mayer, C. Basque, M. Nali, A. Eriks-Brophy, S. D. Soli, and C. Giguère. 2005. Adaptation of the HINT (Hearing in Noise Test) for adult Canadian francophone populations. *International Journal of Audiology* 44(6):358–361.

Valente, M., K. M. Mispagel, J. Tchorz, and D. Fabry. 2006. Effect of type of noise and loudspeaker array on the performance of omnidirectional and directional microphones. *Journal of the American Academy of Audiology* 17(6):398–412.

Vermiglio, A. J. 2008. The American English Hearing in Noise Test. *International Journal of Audiology* 47(6):386–387.

Vermiglio, A. J., S. D. Soli, D. J. Freed, and X. Fang. 2020. The effect of stimulus audibility on the relationship between pure-tone average and speech recognition in noise ability. *Journal of the American Academy of Audiology* 31(3):224–232.

Weiss, D., and J. J. Dempsey. 2008. Performance of bilingual speakers on the English and Spanish versions of the Hearing in Noise Test (HINT). *Journal of the American Academy of Audiology* 19(1):5–17.

Wong, L. L. N., and S. D. Soli. 2005. Development of the Cantonese Hearing in Noise Test (CHINT). *Ear and Hearing* 26(3):276–289.

Wong, L. L. N., S. D. Soli, S. Liu, N. Han, and M. W. Huang. 2007. Development of the Mandarin Hearing in Noise Test (MHINT). *Ear and Hearing* 28(Suppl 2):70S–74S.

4

Characteristics of Hearing and Speech Tests

This chapter focuses on item 2 in the committee's Statement of Task:

Describe the characteristics of hearing tests, administered in the sound field, either binaurally or monaurally, in either quiet or noise, that are in use for those with cochlear implants, and describe to the degree possible:

a. The availability of the selected tests with respect to the instruments themselves, trained administrators of the tests, and insurance coverage or costs incurred with testing;
b. The patient burden of undergoing these tests;
c. Whether testing procedures or parameters, or the appropriateness of the test itself, vary based on the age of the person being tested;
d. Whether the test outcomes are expected to vary based on demographic or other patient characteristic factors, including repeated testing with the same instrument; and
e. The validity, specificity, sensitivity, reliability, and generalizability of the tests.

The committee selected several sentence tests and word tests to describe in this chapter. The tests selected are those that are commonly used to evaluate hearing loss in adults and children with cochlear implants. The chapter begins by addressing a few of the issues in the state of task that are crosscutting, such as test administrators and costs associated with testing. The chapter then discusses the characteristics of each of the following sentence tests and word tests in order of their chronologic development:

Sentence Tests
- Central Institute for the Deaf (CID) Sentences
- City University of New York (CUNY) Sentences
- Hearing in Noise Test (HINT)
- HINT-Children (HINT-C)
- Quick Speech in Noise Test (QuickSIN)
- Bamford-Kowal-Bench Speech in Noise (BKB-SIN)
- Arizona Biomedical (AzBio) Sentences Test
- Pediatric AzBio Sentences Test

Word Tests
- Phonetically Balanced Kindergarten (PBK) Words
- Northwestern University Test No. 6 (NU-6) Words
- Maryland Consonant–Nucleus–Consonant (CNC) Words
- Lexical Neighborhood Test and Multisyllabic Neighborhood Test (LNT and MLNT)
- Words in Noise Test (WIN)
- Digit Triplet Test

The characterizations of individual tests are followed by a section on considerations beyond auditory testing, given that hearing loss affects multiple functional abilities. The information requested in items "a" through "e" above is provided to the degree that is available in the literature. Several of the test characteristics could not be addressed because the information required did not appear to be available in the published literature. Specifically, the committee conducted a literature search on the validity, specificity, sensitivity, reliability, and generalizability of each of the tests described in the chapter. Although committee members found many published papers regarding the reliability of the tests that are summarized in this chapter, they did not find published literature about test validity, specificity, sensitivity, and generalizability. The committee also did not find published literature on outcome variation by patient demographic for all of the tests described. When this information was not available, the committee suggests some patient characteristics that might affect outcomes, based on the committee's professional judgment.

Finally, the chapter provides conclusions and a recommendation based on material covered in Chapters 1 through 4.

CROSS-CUTTING ISSUES

Making decisions about adult cochlear implant candidacy has historically relied heavily on the use of sentence-level speech perception tests. As described in previous chapters, advancements in cochlear implant technology and the resulting improvements in cochlear implant outcomes have necessitated the development and use of increasingly difficult sentence tests over the past several decades.

In the United States, audiologists are the most likely administrators for tests of unaided and aided speech recognition, because those tasks fall within the scope of audiology clinical practice and audiologists are familiar with associated current procedural terminology (CPT) codes for unaided speech audiometry and aided speech recognition. Unaided speech audiometry can be administered and billed solely as a speech reception threshold or SRT (92555), SRT combined with unaided word recognition testing (92556), or both combined with conventional pure-tone audiometry (92557). Assessing aided speech recognition is included under the evaluation of aural rehabilitation status and billed as 92626. Note that CPT 92626 is a time-based code and should not be billed for aided speech recognition assessments lasting less than 31 minutes. For shorter assessments it is recommended that the audiologist bill 92700 (unlisted otorhinolaryngologic service or procedure) and be sure to include appropriate documentation in the clinical report (ASHA, 2020). While there are a number of audiology and otolaryngology practices that are employing audiology technicians, at present technicians are not able to bill for speech audiometry, speech recognition, or the evaluation of aural rehabilitation status. Thus, to ensure compliance with Medicare billing practices, a licensed audiologist should complete the assessments of speech recognition.

In terms of patient burden, the costs of the test are covered by most private and public insurance programs, although patients who are uninsured may face out-of-pocket expenses. From the patient perspective, the burden of completing a sentence or word test is low in terms of time and complexity; however, patients might experience frustration if they realize they cannot accurately understand the test items.

To ensure that test results are not influenced by factors unrelated to perceptual ability, it is important to consider a patient's chronologic age and language level when selecting a particular sentence test. The vocabulary and grammatical structure of test items may be of particular concern; for example, if a child is given a sentence test developed for adults, it might contain many words not in the child's vocabulary so that the score is likely to be lower than if all of the words in the test were known to the child. The vocabulary factor also affects list equivalence if a child has different levels of familiarity with the words within various lists. Test selection must be approached carefully to ensure that the testing is measuring the desired factors (i.e., assessing speech perception abilities) rather than language level. Those same concerns hold for word tests as well.

SENTENCE TESTS

The following sections characterize sentence tests that are commonly used to evaluate hearing loss in adults and children with cochlear implants. The tests are presented in the order of their chronologic development.

Central Institute for the Deaf Sentences

In 1955, Silverman and Hirsh from CID constructed and recorded a set of 100 sentences for use in speech testing (i.e., the CID Sentences). The content and form of the sentences met a set of criteria related to vocabulary and sentence structure laid out by a working group spanning the disciplines of experimental phonetics, linguistics, psychology, and statistics that was hoping to improve the "face validity" of speech testing. Early evaluation of these sentences revealed a close relationship between performance on them and performance on a sample of continuous discourse (Giolas, 1966). The original CID Sentences were revised by Harris and colleagues in 1961 in an attempt to provide greater homogeneity of sentence length and were afterwards known as the Revised CID Sentence Lists.

Availability

The CID Everyday Speech Sentences are available for purchase from Oaktree Products.

Reliability

Giolas and Duffy (1973) investigated the equivalency of scores obtained with the original and revised lists. As part of this work, high-quality master tapes were made of all sentences (10 lists of 10 sentences for each version of the test) being spoken by one male talker with a general American accent. The recordings were distorted using low-pass filtering at 420 Hz to produce a sufficient number of error responses to allow for list comparisons. The results strongly suggested that under the study's test conditions none of the lists within the original or revised CID sentences could be considered to be equivalent for most testing purposes.

City University of New York Sentences

As originally developed, the CUNY Sentences consist of 48 sets of 12 topic-related sentences where all sentences within a set relate to the same topic. Each set consists of four statements, four questions, and four commands (Boothroyd et al., 1985). Sentence length varies from 3 to 14 words.

Availability

The CUNY Sentences are available for purchase from Auditec, Inc.

Reliability

To determine the reliability and equivalency of the original 48 sentence sets, nine adults with normal hearing were provided visual-only information from recordings of a woman producing the sentences, supplemental audio information containing only fundamental frequency information, and the topic of the sentence (Boothroyd et al., 1985). Listeners were inexperienced lipreaders. Their task was to repeat as much of each sentence as possible. For the given recording and test conditions, the CUNY sentence sets were found to be of equivalent difficulty. However, short-term leaning effects were present as revealed by improving scores over the first eight or nine sets of sentences. The 95% confidence intervals of a single score of approximately 85 percent was assumed to be +/− 16 percentage points, excluding the short-term learning effect described above. It is important to note that the apparent learning effects may have been due to improvements in lipreading performance, improvements in the ability to integrate limited acoustic information with visual information, or increased familiarity of the task.

Hearing in Noise Test

The HINT, described in detail in Chapter 3, was developed by Nilsson et al. (1994) as a measure of sentence speech reception thresholds. The HINT makes use of modified BKB sentences (Bench et al., 1979), which were originally constructed for use with British children. These sentences contain common nouns and verbs found in transcriptions of children's speech and were designed to be scored based on the recognition of key words. Modifications included removing British idioms but maintaining the same sentence length. Great care was taken to match the phonemic content of the 25 10-sentence-long lists.

Availability

To verify the availability of the HINT, the committee corresponded with three individuals at Natus, a company that produces, among other products, medical equipment used in the diagnosis of hearing loss. Natus previously distributed the HINT Pro System, an audiometer used for assessing hearing, which contained a library of all of the various versions of the HINT. The committee learned that this system is no longer produced and that the HINT is not otherwise available for stand-alone purchase. In addition, it is not accessible for many patients (see Chapter 3). While it is true that a number of long-established cochlear implant clinics may still possess a copy of the HINT, those clinics are not necessarily geographically dispersed. This means that individuals might need to travel hundreds of miles in order to find an audiologist who is capable of offering the HINT, greatly increasing patient burden in terms of time and cost.

Reliability

Test validation studies confirmed that reliable sentence-level speech reception thresholds can be obtained in quiet and in noise with adaptive procedures using the HINT's short lists of brief sentences. Confidence intervals (CIs) suggest that the use of one 10-sentence list per condition makes it possible to detect differences of 2.98 dB (decibels) in quiet and 2.41 dB in noise. CIs improve as the number of sentence lists increases. The reliability of sentence speech reception thresholds was also found to vary as a function of bandwidth, but was only substantially degraded when the bandwidth dropped below about 2,000 Hz,[1] suggesting that the test is fairly robust to the variations in audibility associated with hearing loss and personal sensory devices. While variability is greater in listeners with hearing loss, the reliability of the test in these listeners is still quite close to that measured in listeners with normal hearing (Gilbert et al., 2013; Robson, 2001; Schafer, 2010).

The HINT sentence lists are intended for adaptive measures of speech reception thresholds. The popular use of these sentences in the evaluation of cochlear implant patients disregards this intent in that the sentences are presented at fixed levels in quiet or in the presence of fixed-level noise. Because of that, the reliability demonstrated during initial test construction does not necessarily apply to the common use of these sentences with cochlear implant users.

---

[1] The hertz (Hz) is the derived unit of frequency in the International System of Units and is defined as one cycle per second.

Hearing in Noise Test-Children

The HINT-C is composed of a subset of sentences from the HINT that could be accurately identified by a group of 5- and 6-year-old children. In total there are 10 lists of 10 sentences each for use in adaptive threshold testing in quiet or in noise.

Availability

The HINT-C is no longer available for purchase by cochlear implant audiologists or others (see HINT availability).

Reliability

Given that the HINT-C is composed of a subset of sentences from the HINT, reliability is expected to be similar between the two tests. Performance on the HINT-C is age-dependent. Specifically, 6- to 12-year-old children have been shown to perform significantly more poorly than older children and adults (Nilsson et al., 1996; Schafer, 2010).

Quick Speech in Noise Test

In 2004, Killion et al. (2004) developed a shorted and improved version of the SIN test (Etymōtic Research, 1993), which they named the QuickSIN test. The original SIN test uses 360 Institute of Electrical and Electronics Engineers (IEEE) sentences (Rothauser, 1969) as target speech and four-talker babble (Auditec of St. Louis, 1971) as "noise." Each sentence is scored on five key words, with partial credit available for partially correct answers; however, inter-observer reliability of partial credit scoring has been found to be low (Bentler, 2000). While the original IEEE sentences lists were phonetically balanced, these balanced groupings were not maintained in the SIN test. Another concern about the SIN test is that Bentler (2000) demonstrated that it suffered from both ceiling and floor effects. The updated QuickSIN test uses a significantly smaller number of the original SIN's IEEE sentences (a total of 72), which were carefully selected to ensure a balancing of lists, and it does not allow for partial credit scoring. The QuickSIN is composed of 12 equivalent lists, each containing 6 different IEEE sentences. A single sentence (as opposed to five sentences in the SIN test) is presented at each of six decreasing signal-to-noise ratios (SNRs) between successive sentences (from 25 to 0 dB SNR, in 5 dB steps). The listener's score is calculated as the SNR the listener requires to understand 50 percent of the sentences' key words. As its name implies, the QuickSIN is fast to administer, with each list taking approximately 1 minute to complete, compared with 6 minutes for a single SIN test block.

Availability

The QuickSIN Test is available for purchase from Etymōtic Research.

Reliability

The QuickSIN's 12 equivalent lists have a standard deviation of 1.4 dB for SRN estimation when a single list is administered, which is slightly better than what would have been expected based on the SIN test, an improvement that is likely due to the more careful selection of sentences for the QuickSIN. In terms of reliability, a single QuickSIN list is accurate to ± 2.2 dB at the 80% CI (2.7 dB for a 95% CI), which the authors suggest is adequate for clinical testing. Reliability improves when more than one list is administered. For example, averaging two lists increases accuracy to from ± 2.2 dB to ± 1.6 dB for an 80% CI (and from ± 2.7 to ± 1.9 dB for a 95% CI). When comparing two conditions, the use of multiple QuickSIN lists is important. For example, when using only one list per condition, results would have to be greater than 3.2 dB to be considered statistically different, given an 80% CI; that difference score decreases to 2.2 dB for two lists, to 1.8 dB for three lists, with further, diminishing decreases as the number of test lists continues to increase.

Bamford-Kowal-Bench Speech in Noise

The BKB-SIN test is a sentence test that was developed primarily for use with both children and patients who are candidates for or already have cochlear implants (Etymōtic Research, 2005). Like the HINT, it uses Americanized BKB sentences that are short, highly redundant, rich with semantic and syntax context cues, and at a first-grade reading level. The main differences between the HINT and the BKB-SIN are the methods used to determine the 50 percent point and the type of background noise. While the HINT uses a modified adaptive procedure that brackets the 50 percent point, the BKB-SIN, like QuickSIN and the WIN (described below), relies on a descending level of noise and the Spearman-Karber equation to calculate the 50 percent point.

The BKB-SIN, when presented in quiet at 70 dB SPL, is the standard test for evaluating candidacy for adult cochlear implantation in the United Kingdom (NICE, 2019). BKB-SIN sentences are also used after implantation to demonstrate improvement (Cullington and Aidi, 2017). The BKB sentences used in the BKB-SIN and the HINT provide more semantic context than the IEEE sentences used in the QuickSIN (Wilson et al., 2007). Thus, better recognition scores should be expected on the BKB-SIN and the HINT than on the QuickSIN and the WIN.

Availability

The BKB-SIN test can be purchased from Auditec, Inc., and Etymōtic Research.

Reliability

The reliability of the BKB-SIN is related to the number of test items, age, and cochlear implant use. The largest increase in reliability by incremental increases in the number of lists is observed between the use of one versus two lists (0.5 dB for adults with normal hearing, 0.9 dB for adult cochlear implant users, 1.2 dB for 5–6-year-olds, 0.7 dB for 7–10-year-olds, and 0.7 for 11–14-year-olds), which adds just 3 minutes to testing. The test manual provides information regarding the magnitude of difference that can be reliably measured when comparing two conditions as a function of number of lists for adults with normal hearing, adult cochlear implant users, and children.

Arizona Biomedical Sentences Test

The AzBio Sentences Test was devised by Spahr and Dorman at Arizona State University specifically as an experiment to compare the speech understanding abilities of high-performing patients implanted with different cochlear implant systems, in everyday listening environments (Spahr and Dorman, 2005; Spahr et al., 2007). The relatively complex sentences within each list are spoken by four different talkers using a conversational speaking style and rate, which allows for an estimation of real-life performance.

In 2008, Gifford and colleagues applied the tests more generally to evaluate the speech perception abilities of hearing impaired people with cochlear implants. They reported that the AzBio test produced results that were highly correlated with monosyllabic word scores and did not suffer the same ceiling effects in quiet as other sentence tests (ceiling effects are observed when subjects consistently score at or near 100 percent, such that any further improvement is unable to be detected). Ceiling effects are minimized in quiet and in noise because the materials are more difficult than the HINT sentences (Gifford et al., 2008; Spahr et al., 2012). Fabry et al. (2009) agreed with that assessment and suggested that AzBio sentences could be of value in evaluating hearing in cochlear implant users, both pre- and post-implant. Cochlear implant manufacturers have thus moved to include AzBio sentence lists in a new battery of tests that will serve as the standard for assessing pre- and post-implant hearing.

Availability

The AzBio Sentences Test can be purchased from Auditory Potential, LLC.

Reliability

In 2012, Spahr et al. (2012) set out to create and validate a new set of sentence tests to add to the AzBio sentence corpus. Four talkers, two male and two female, were selected to each record 250 sentences. The Spahr et al. (2012) validation study found that 29 of the 33 lists of sentences yielded scores that, when averaged over the 15 cochlear implant users tested, were not statistically different from one another. However, individual listeners demonstrated considerable variability in performance across lists. The researchers chose 15 of the 29 lists to include in the AzBio Sentences Test. They noted that the test had not been validated for children and that further research would need to be conducted to assess the reliability of the sentences for specific populations.

Pediatric Arizona Biomedical Sentences Test

The popularity of the original AzBio test resulted in clinicians using these materials with their pediatric patients. Concerns regarding the appropriateness of the content of some of these sentences, paired with the fact that the test was too difficult for some poorer-performing adult cochlear implant users, led to the creation of a new set of materials. The validated Pediatric AzBio Sentences Test consists of 16 equivalent lists of 20 sentences spoken by a single female talker (Spahr et al., 2014).

Availability

The Pediatric AzBio Sentences Test can be purchased from Auditory Potential, LLC.

Reliability

Spahr et al. (2014) created recordings of 450 sentences (3–12 words in length) that had been generated by 5- to 12-year-old children, with and without hearing loss, during everyday conversations. All of the sentences were recorded by one female talker and screened for inclusion by presenting them to 30 kindergarten and first-grade children with normal hearing. Following a sentence intelligibility estimation procedure in which adults listened to versions of the sentences that had processed through a 15-channel noiseband vocoder, a type of filtering that produces a signal that contains the same kind of speech information available to a cochlear implant user, a total of 320 sentences were chosen and divided into 16 lists of 20 sentences each. The mean list intelligibility per list was 78.6 percent correct. The equivalency of these pre-assigned lists was validated by a group of experienced adult cochlear implant users and pediatric hearing aid and cochlear implant users. The performance achieved by adult and pediatric cochlear implant users averaged 74 percent correct and 77 percent correct, respectively. Statistical analysis revealed no significant differences across lists. The authors provide CIs for the administration of one list per condition and two lists per condition that are based on methods originally described by Thornton and Raffin (1978). The availability of 16 equivalent lists provides the opportunity to assess changes in performance across conditions over time.

WORD TESTS

The section above highlighted the sentence tests that have been developed and can be used for individuals with cochlear implants. This section will focus on word tests.

Phonetically Balanced Kindergarten Words

The PBK test (Haskins, 1949) was the product of the unpublished master's thesis work of Harriet Haskins. While four test lists were generated originally, only three of the lists have been used clinically because the fourth list (List 2 in the original work) did not produce results equivalent to the other three. At the time they were chosen for the PBK test, the test words were all found within the 2,500 words of highest frequency spoken by preschool children (IKU, 1928). However, it is likely that today's very young children with hearing loss may be unfamiliar with a number of the words contained within the PBK lists (Kirk et al., 1995; Meyer and Pisoni, 1999). In this open-set test of monosyllabic word understanding, children are asked to repeat back words presented to them without any visual cues.

Availability

The PBK test can be purchased from Auditec, Inc.

Reliability

Haskins collected speech perception data from adults with normal hearing listening to the PBK lists. It was during this testing that List 2 was identified as being more audible than the other lists. For this reason, only Lists 1, 3, and 4 from the original thesis work are used in clinical practice. Meyer and Pisoni (1999) were unable to find evidence that either children or listeners with hearing loss were tested when the reliability of these word lists was evaluated. In their own work, Meyer and Pisoni (1999) found that the mean frequency of words from List 2 was higher than the mean frequency of words from the other lists, which likely accounts for them as having been described as "more audible" in Haskins's thesis. These authors also found that the ratio of the frequency of the stimulus to the density of the lexical neighborhood was more favorable for the words in List 2 than for the words in the other lists. Finally, findings of Kluck et al. (1997) suggest there will be age effects on the PBK test that may be related to word familiarity. Specifically, they found that 4-year-old children with normal hearing performed at near ceiling levels on the PBK test, while 3-year-old children performed slightly lower. The investigators also asked the parents of those 3- and 4-year-olds to judge whether their children were familiar with each of the PBK words. Results suggested that the words were slightly less familiar to the 3-year-olds but that, overall, most words on the PBK test were familiar to the general population of preschool age children.

Northwestern University Test No. 6 Words

The NU-6 test was first described in 1966 by Tillman and Carhart. This test contains four lists of 50 CNC monosyllabic words. The authors took great care to preserve the phonemic distribution of the pool of 1,263 words initially selected by Lehiste and Peterson (1959), who recommended that each initial, medial, and final phoneme appears in a single list of 50 words with the same relative frequency as found in the total pool of words.

Availability

The NU-6 test can be purchased from Auditec, Inc.

Reliability

Experiments conducted with 40 listeners with normal hearing and 12 listeners with hearing loss suggest both good inter-list equivalence and high test–retest reliability. For both groups of subjects, the maximum test–retest difference was always less than 10 percent (five words) and almost always (i.e., 92 percent of the time) within 6 percent (three words).

Maryland Consonant–Nucleus–Consonant Words

The Maryland CNC Words test is routinely used in U.S. Department of Veterans Affairs medical centers as part of the audiological Compensation and Pension exam, which determines hearing disability related to military service (Mendel et al., 2014). Causey et al. (1984) used Peterson and Lehiste's revised CNC words lists (Peterson and Lehiste, 1962) to develop this open-set, monosyllabic CNC test. Recordings were made by one male talker speaking the test words within the phrase "Say the [test word] again."

Availability

The Maryland CNC Words test is available for order from Richard Wilson at Arizona State University.

Reliability

Causey et al. (1984) examined list equivalency by presenting all lists to a total of 40 male veterans with sensorineural hearing loss, 10 listeners per group, with each group assigned to listen at 20, 30, 40, or 44 dB sound level (SL) in relation to their speech reception thresholds. Results suggested that 6 of the 10 available lists produced equivalent scores (i.e., Lists 1, 3, 6, 7, 9, and 10). Performance across those lists varied by a range of only 3.6 percent.

Test–retest reliability was examined in 10 listeners who were tested twice with an average span of 4 weeks between test sessions. They listened at a 44 dB sensation level. The differences in average scores between the two test sessions were never greater than 5.6 percent. The correlations between test sessions were significant for all 10 lists, with the strongest correlation between List 1 and List 2. When evaluated using Thornton and Raffin's (1978) 95 percent critical different values for a 50-item test, only one listener showed a significant difference across the two test sessions and, then, only for List 2. Based on both of these experiences, the developers suggested using the six equivalent and reliable lists when assessing speech perception abilities.

Lexical Neighborhood Test and Multisyllabic Neighborhood Test

Given that both word frequency and lexical similarity affect speech understanding, Kirk et al. (1995) set out to develop new word recognition tests, one monosyllabic (the LNT) and one multisyllabic (the MLNT), in which the lexical properties of the test items were carefully controlled. They used a measure of lexical similarity that considered the number of "neighbors," or words that differed by just one phoneme from a target word. The frequency of a word combined with its "density" within a lexical neighborhood can be used to sort words into dense neighborhoods (i.e., words that have many lexical neighbors) and sparse neighborhoods (i.e., words with few lexical neighbors). Words can be further classified from a scale of "easy" (with the easiest being high-frequency words from sparse neighborhoods) to "hard" (with the hardest being low-frequency words from dense neighborhoods).

Test stimulus words were drawn from Logan's (1992) analysis of a sample of child language obtained from the Child Language Data Exchange System database (MacWhinney and Snow, 1985). Specifically, words produced by 3- to 5-year-old children were selected and sorted into four lists, each composed of 25 monosyllables for the LNT and 25 two- or three-syllable words for the MLNT. Two of the word lists for each of these tests were lexically easy, and two were lexically hard. While now available as recorded lists, during the initial development and testing, the words were presented via monitored live voice to a group of pediatric cochlear implant users. The analysis of this testing revealed that young cochlear implant users were sensitive to the acoustic–phonetic similarity among the LNT's words in that they performed better with the easy lists than with the hard lists. Furthermore, word recognition scores were higher for multisyllabic than monosyllabic words for both easy and hard lists. In addition to information about speech perception ability, the LNT and the MLNT allow for an examination of the perceptual processes underlying spoken word recognition and may also be used to better understand the organization of sound patterns of words in young children's lexicons and the processes used to access these patterns.

Availability

The LNT and the MLNT can be purchased from Auditec, Inc.

Reliability

As a follow-up to the initial development and testing of the LNT and the MLNT lists, Kirk et al. (1999) investigated the reliability and inter-list equivalency of recordings of these lists. Their results showed that even with recorded presentations, performance was better on easy lists than hard ones, there were no differences between matched lists, and test–retest reliability was high. High reliability was demonstrated in two ways: (1) no difference in LNT and MLNT scores over separate test sessions and (2) strong correlations ($r \geq 0.83$) between test sessions.

Words in Noise Test

The WIN was developed by Wilson et al. (2003) to provide a test that would qualify speech understanding in multi-talker babble in terms of hearing loss for speech, expressed in terms of signal-to-babble ratio (S/B) loss. The resultant instrument presents 10 NU-6 words (described above) spoken by a female talker (Tillman and Carhart, 1966) at each of seven S/Bs, in 4 dB steps from 0 to 24 dB, with the babble being comprised of three male and three female talkers speaking about various topics. The use of monosyllabic words in the WIN provides a good measure of basic auditory function because the effect of memory and linguistic context on recognition are minimized. Additionally, monosyllabic words recorded in isolation decrease the chance of blurring phoneme boundaries with co-articulation (Wilson et al., 2007).

Availability

The WIN is available for order from Richard Wilson at Arizona State University.

Reliability

The WIN is sensitive to the presence of even high-frequency hearing loss. The 90th percentile for listeners with normal hearing was observed to be 6 dB S/B. Based on this observation, any test outcome suggesting a S/B ratio greater than 6 dB is considered an abnormal finding. Even though all listeners with hearing loss who participated in experiments to develop and evaluate the WIN test had monosyllabic word understanding abilities equal to or greater than 80 percent correct in quiet (mean 89 percent), more than 95 percent of them had abnormal WIN scores. Mean data revealed a 6–9 dB difference in the 50 percent points for listeners with normal hearing and hearing loss, which is consistent with findings obtained by others (Dubno et al., 1984; Tillman et al., 1970; Wilson and Strouse, 2002) who have examined the speech perception in noise abilities of these two groups of listeners.

Digit Triplet Test

Smits et al. (2004) developed a speech-in-noise test for use as an objective, self-test for hearing loss in Dutch listeners. They made the fully automated test controllable by a computer and available for taking over the telephone. In approximately 3 minutes, the test can produce a speech reception threshold using an adaptive approach based on the perception of 20 strings of 3 single digits (a total of 23 strings are chosen randomly from a body of 80 triplets), spoken by a female talker and presented in a background of speech-shaped noise (matched in long-term average spectrum to the digits), which is not affected by telephone type or listening environment.

It is becoming increasingly common to measure speech understanding with numerical digits. This type of testing has an advantage compared with sentence tests in that it does not rely on the listener's cognitive ability to recognize contextual cues and limited language ability does not impede testing as much with other tests (Cullington and Aidi, 2017). Digit triplet testing is also easier than sentence tests to conduct over the phone or the Internet or to self-administer (Leensen et al., 2011; Smits and Houtgast, 2005; Smits et al., 2006; Watson et al., 2012). The digit triplet test also minimizes lexical knowledge, which can be useful for non-native speakers of English (Ramkissoon et al., 2002). Testing digit triplets in noise has been used to screen hearing in hundreds of thousands of people worldwide (Stam et al., 2015; Williams-Sanchez et al., 2014). It has also been used successfully with both adults and children with cochlear implants (Kaandorp et al., 2015; Mishra et al., 2015), its results correlate well with those of a sentence test in noise, and it has been shown in at least one Dutch study to have adequate repeatability (Kaandorp et al., 2015).

Availability

Availability in the United States is unknown.

Reliability

The digit triplet test is highly reliable, as evidenced by its measurement error of less than 1 dB (i.e., standard deviation of repeated measurements within subjects). This high level of reliability is observed in the controlled conditions of audiology clinics as well as in listeners' homes. Using a standard of a sentence speech reception threshold test (Plomp and Mimpen, 1979) administered via headphone, the sensitivity and specificity of the digit triplet are 0.91 and 0.93, respectively, which the authors cite as evidence of its utility for screening purposes. A digit triplet SNR of –4.1 dB serves as the cut-off for normal and impaired hearing.

Table 4-1 presents a summary table of the information provided in this chapter on the individual tests.

CONSIDERATIONS BEYOND AUDITORY TESTING

Auditory testing, including both audiometric thresholds and speech testing, is considered the gold standard of assessing auditory function in individuals with hearing loss. Cochlear implant candidacy and outcomes

TABLE 4-1 Reliability and Other Notable Characteristics of Selected Sentence and Word Tests

Test	Year of Publication	Target Population	Reliability and Other Notable Characteristics
Sentence Tests			
Central Institute for the Deaf (CID) Sentences	1955	Adults	Low reliability: individual test lists do not produce equivalent scores.
City University of New York (CUNY) Sentences	1985	Adults	Sentence lists are of equivalent difficulty.
Hearing in Noise Test (HINT)	1994	Adults	Use of one test list is capable of detecting differences in reception thresholds for sentences of 2.98 decibels (dB) in quiet and 2.41 dB in noise. Confidence intervals improve as the number of sentence lists increases. When used with listeners with hearing loss, reliability is quite close to that demonstrated for listeners with normal hearing. Note: This reliability information is for results obtained with the HINT administered as intended by the test authors. Use of the HINT with cochlear implant users almost always deviates from these procedures. Availability is limited as the test is no longer sold.
HINT-Children (HINT-C)	1996	Children	Reliability is similar to that of the HINT. Younger children (i.e., 6–12 years of age) perform significantly poorer than older children and adults. Availability is limited as the test is no longer sold.
Quick Speech in Noise Test (QuickSIN)	2004	Adults	Each of the test's 12 lists produce equivalent scores. A single list is accurate to ± 2.2. dB (80% confidence interval) and to ± 2.7 dB (95% confidence interval). Reliability improves as the number of lists administered increases.

continued

TABLE 4-1 Continued

Test	Year of Publication	Target Population	Reliability and Other Notable Characteristics
Bamford-Kowal-Bench Speech in Noise (BKB-SIN) Test	2005	Children and cochlear implant candidates and users	Reliability of the BKB-SIN is related to the number of test items, age, and cochlear implant use. Largest gains in reliability are obtained with a move from administration of one list to two lists.
Arizona Biomedical (AzBio) Sentences Test	2005	Adults	The 15 lists of sentences available in the AzBio test produce equivalent results.
Pediatric Arizona Biomedical (AzBio) Sentences Test	2014	Children	The AzBio test lists produce equivalent scores. Confidence intervals are provided for the administration of one and two sentence lists per test condition and are based on the methods of Thornton and Raffin (1978).
Phonetically Balanced Kindergarten (PBK) Words	1949	Children	Of the original four PBK sentences lists, Lists 1, 3, and 4 have been found to be equivalent. These are the lists used in clinical practice.

Word Tests

Test	Year of Publication	Target Population	Reliability and Other Notable Characteristics
Northwestern University Test No. 6 (NU-6) Words	1966	Adults	Testing with listeners with normal hearing and listeners with hearing loss have revealed good inter-list equivalence and high test–retest reliability.
Maryland CNC Words	1984	Adults	The test offers six equivalent and reliable lists.
Lexical Neighborhood Test (LNT)	1995	Children	High reliability on the LNT and the MLNT has been demonstrated in excellent test–retest reliability and strong correlations between test sessions. The tests' matched lists provide equivalent performance.
Multisyllabic Neighborhood Test (MLNT)	1995	Children	
Words in Noise Test (WIN)	2003	Adults	The WIN is sensitive to the presence of hearing loss, even just high-frequency hearing loss. A signal-to-babble ratio greater than 6 dB on this test is an abnormal finding.
Digit Triplet	2004	Adults	This test uses numerical digits rather than words. It is a highly reliable test as evidenced by a measurement error of less than 1 dB. Reliability is equivalent for tests administered in audiology clinics as well as in private homes. Availability in the United States is unknown.

are often determined based on a defined performance level obtained from auditory testing. As described in this chapter, there are many different speech tests available that can be used in specific patient populations. However, hearing loss can have impacts beyond what is captured during auditory testing. Many studies have shown that significant hearing loss can affect emotional, social, academic, and occupational elements of life. Additionally, there is evidence to suggest that measurements of speech recognition tests do not always correlate with subjective perception of auditory performance (e.g., Bentler, 2005; Wackym et al., 2007).

The consequence of hearing loss on quality of life in cochlear implant users can be measured using self-report questionnaires, such as two versions of the Cochlear Implant Quality of Life (McRackan et al., 2019), the Cochlear Implant Function Index (Coelho et al., 2009), and the Nijmegen Cochlear Implant Questionnaire (Hinderink et al., 2000). These are questionnaires that have been specifically designed for use in the cochlear implant population. There are also many questionnaires that exist that can provide an assessment of hearing handicap, perceived disability, or listening effort. Some examples include the Hearing Handicap Inventory for Adults/Elderly (Newman et al., 1990; Ventry and Weinstein, 1982), the Communication Profile for the Hearing Impaired (Demorest and Erdman, 1987), the Abbreviated Profile of Hearing Aid Benefit (Cox and Alexander, 1995), and the Speech, Spatial and Qualities of Hearing Scale (Gatehouse and Noble, 2004).

Questionnaires are available that can be completed by parents of young children or by clinicians to supplement audiological test results and provide important information regarding a child's auditory skills. Examples of questionnaires available for use with young children with hearing loss include the LittlEars (Weichbold et al., 2005), the Infant–Toddler version of the Meaningful Auditory Integration Scale (Zimmerman-Phillips et al., 2000), and the Auditory Skills Checklist (Meinzen-Derr et al., 2007). Examples of questionnaires designed for use with children with hearing loss over the age of 3 years include the Meaningful Auditory Integration Scale (Robbins et al., 1991), the Parents' Evaluation of Aural/Oral Performance of Children (Ching and Hill, 2007), and the Auditory Skills Checklist (Meinzen-Derr et al., 2007).

To fully evaluate auditory function, it can be helpful to include the subjective perspective from the patient or from their parent. Self-report or parent-report measurements, when used as a supplement to auditory threshold and speech testing, can help capture the complete picture of the impact of hearing loss in a given individual.

CONCLUSIONS AND RECOMMENDATION

As discussed in Chapter 3, the HINT has several limitations in its characteristics and deviation from its intended use (i.e., the use of a single male speaker and speech-spectrum background noise, and administration in quiet or fixed noise presentation rather than its intended adaptive design). Furthermore, the Minimum Speech Test Battery (MSTB) recommendations note that "advances in technology, improvements in outcomes, and changes in candidacy criteria have resulted in ceiling effects on the HINT sentences when presented in quiet" (Gifford et al., 2008, 2010; MSTB, 2011). U.S. Food and Drug Administration usage in effectiveness studies and unclear candidacy criteria from insurance providers (e.g., Centers for Medicare & Medicaid Services) add to the limitations of the test. Finally, due to its exclusion from the most recent MSTB and the fact that it is no longer available for purchase, the HINT is difficult for clinics across the United States to obtain.

Overall, the HINT has been widely used to measure cochlear implant candidacy and post-operative outcomes since its inception in 1994. However, the test characteristics, the state of cochlear implant technology, and the environment that made the HINT a common choice of assessment in 1994 are different in 2021.

Word recognition testing as employed in most audiology clinics includes administration of a phonemically balanced word list such as the NU-6 (Tillman and Carhart, 1966), CID W-22 (Silverman and Hirsh, 1955), or the Maryland CNC (Causey et al., 1984) word lists. Monosyllabic word recognition is currently an accepted measure for determining U.S. Social Security Administration (SSA) disability as related to hearing loss for individuals without cochlear implants. Monosyllabic word recognition is currently the standard for pediatric cochlear implant candidacy, and the field is moving toward use of a monosyllabic word recognition criterion for determining adult candidacy in the United States (e.g., Buchman et al., 2020). Additionally, monosyllabic word recognition has been used to characterize post-operative outcomes for both adult and pediatric cochlear implant recipients for more than two decades (MSTB, 2011). Furthermore, SSA has been using monosyllabic words to determine initial and continued eligibility for SSA benefits for individuals with hearing loss not treated with cochlear implantation. For those reasons, the committee recommends monosyllabic word tests, rather than sentence tests.

Given the limitations of the Hearing in Noise Test, the committee recommends the use of a monosyllabic word recognition test to assess hearing loss in individuals treated with cochlear implantation, consistent with what the U.S. Social Security Administration currently uses

to determine disability in adults and children with hearing loss not treated with cochlear implantation. Administration of the word test should include a full word list that is standardized and phonetically or phonemically balanced.

The committee believes that is the direction that SSA should be adopting for assessment of cochlear implant recipients. Chapter 6 provides more specific recommendations for characteristics of hearing tests that should be used to assess hearing loss in individuals with cochlear implants.

REFERENCES

ASHA (American Speech–Language–Hearing Association). 2020. *Medicare fee schedule for audiologists*. https://www.asha.org/siteassets/uploadedfiles/2020-Medicare-Physician-Fee-Schedule-Audiology.pdf (accessed October 17, 2020).
Auditec of St. Louis. 1971. *Four-talker babble*. St. Louis, MO: Auditec of St. Louis.
Bench, J., A. Kowal, and J. Bamford. 1979. The BKB (Bamford-Kowal-Bench) sentence lists for partially-hearing children. *British Journal of Audiology* 13(3):108–112.
Bentler, R. A. 2000. List equivalency and test–retest reliability of the Speech in Noise test. *American Journal of Audiology* 9(2):84–100.
Bentler, R. A. 2005. Effectiveness of directional microphones and noise reduction schemes in hearing aids: A systematic review of the evidence. *Journal of the American Academy of Audiology* 16(7):473–484.
Boothroyd, A., L. Hanin, and T. Hnath. 1985. *A sentence test of speech perception: Reliability, set equivalence, and short-term learning*. City University of New York Internal Report. https://academicworks.cuny.edu/gc_pubs/399 (accessed January 16, 2021).
Causey, G. D., L. J. Hood, C. L. Hermanson, and L. S. Bowling. 1984. The Maryland CNC test: Normative studies. *International Journal of Audiology* 23(6):552–568.
Ching, T. Y. C., and M. Hill. 2007. The Parents' Evaluation of Aural/Oral Performance of Children (PEACH) scale: Normative data. *Journal of the American Academy of Audiology* 18(3):220–235.
Coelho, D. H., P. E. Hammerschlag, Y. Bat-Chava, and D. Kohan. 2009. Psychometric validity of the Cochlear Implant Function Index (CIFI): A quality of life assessment tool for adult cochlear implant users. *Cochlear Implants International* 10(2):70–83.
Cox, R. M., and G. C. Alexander. 1995. The abbreviated profile of hearing aid benefit. *Ear and Hearing* 16(2):176–186.
Cullington, H. E., and T. Aidi. 2017. Is the digit triplet test an effective and acceptable way to assess speech recognition in adults using cochlear implants in a home environment? *Cochlear Implants International* 18(2):97–105.
Demorest, M. E., and S. A. Erdman. 1987. Development of the Communication Profile for the Hearing Impaired. *Journal of Speech and Hearing Disorders* 52(2):129–143.
Dubno, J. R., D. D. Dirks, and D. E. Morgan. 1984. Effects of age and mild hearing loss on speech recognition in noise. *Journal of the Acoustical Society of America* 76(1):87–96.
Etymōtic Research. 1993. *The SIN test*. Elk Grove, IL: Etymōtic Research.
Etymōtic Research. 2005. *BKB–SIN user's manual*. https://www.etymotic.com/downloads/dl/file/id/260/product/160/bkb_sintm_user_manual.pdf (accessed October 17, 2020).
Fabry, D., J. Firszt, R. Gifford, L. Holden, and D. Koch. 2009. Evaluating speech perception benefit in adult cochlear implant recipients. *Audiology Today* 21(3):36–43.

Gatehouse, S., and I. Noble. 2004. The Speech, Spatial and Qualities of Hearing Scale (SSQ). *International Journal of Audiology* 43(2):85–99.

Gifford, R. H., J. K. Shallop, and A. M. Peterson. 2008. Speech recognition materials and ceiling effects: Considerations for cochlear implant programs. *Audiology and Neurotology* 13(3):193–205.

Gilbert, J. L., T. N. Tamati, and D. B. Pisoni. 2013. Development, reliability, and validity of PRESTO: A new high-variability sentence recognition test. *Journal of the American Academy of Audiology* 24(1):26–36.

Giolas, T. 1966. Comparative intelligibility scores of sentence lists and continuous discourse. *Journal of Auditory Research* 6:31–38.

Giolas, T. G., and J. R. Duffy. 1973. Equivalency of CID and revised CID sentence lists. *Journal of Speech and Hearing Research* 16(4):549–555.

Haskins, H. 1949. *A phonetically balanced test of speech discrimination for children*. Evanston, IL: Northwestern University.

Hinderink, J. B., P. F. M. Krabbe, and P. Van Den Broek. 2000. Development and application of a health-related quality-of-life instrument for adults with cochlear implants: The Nijmegen Cochlear Implant Questionnaire. *Otolaryngology—Head and Neck Surgery* 123(6):756–765.

IKU (International Kindergarten Union Child Study Committee). 1928. *A study of the vocabulary of children before entering the first grade*. Washington, DC: International Kindergarten Union.

Kaandorp, M. W., C. Smits, P. Merkus, S. T. Goverts, and J. M. Festen. 2015. Assessing speech recognition abilities with digits in noise in cochlear implant and hearing aid users. *International Journal of Audiology* 54(1):48–57.

Killion, M. C., P. A. Niquette, G. I. Gudmundsen, L. J. Revit, and S. Banerjee. 2004. Development of a Quick Speech-in-Noise test for measuring signal-to-noise ratio loss in normal-hearing and hearing-impaired listeners. *Journal of the Acoustical Society of America* 116(4 I):2395–2405.

Kirk, K. I., D. B. Pisoni, and M. J. Osberger. 1995. Lexical effects on spoken word recognition by pediatric cochlear implant users. *Ear and Hearing* 16(5):470–481.

Kirk, K. I., L. S. Eisenberg, A. S. Martinez, and M. Hay-McCutcheon. 1999. Lexical neighborhood test: Test–retest reliability and interlist equivalency. *Journal of the American Academy of Audiology* 10(3):113–123.

Kluck, M., D. Pisoni, and K. Kirk. 1997. Performance of normal-hearing children on open-set speech perception tests. In H. C. Nusbaum, D. B. Pisoni, and C. K. Davis (eds.), *Research on spoken language processing, report no. 21*. Bloomington, IN: Speech Research Laboratory. Pp. 349–366.

Leensen, M. C. J., J. A. P. M. De Laat, and W. A. Dreschler. 2011. Speech-in-noise screening tests by internet, part 1: Test evaluation for noise-induced hearing loss identification. *International Journal of Audiology* 50(11):823–834.

Lehiste, I., and G. E. Peterson. 1959. Linguistic considerations in the study of speech intelligibility. *Journal of the Acoustical Society of America* 31(3):280–286.

Logan, J. S. 1992. *A computational analysis of young children's lexicons*. Bloomington, IN: Indiana University Press.

MacWhinney, B., and C. Snow. 1985. The child language data exchange system. *Journal of Child Language* 12(2):271–295.

McRackan, T. R., B. N. Hand, C. A. Velozo, J. R. Dubno, J. S. Golub, E. P. Wilkinson, D. Mills, J. P. Carey, N. Vorasubin, V. Brunk, M. L. Carlson, C. L. Driscoll, D. P. Sladen, E. L. Camposeo, M. A. Holcomb, P. R. Lambert, T. A. Meyer, C. Thomas, A. C. Moberly, N. H. Blevins, J. B. Larky, R. P. Herzano, M. E. Hoffer, S. M. Prentiss, R. N. Samy, S. P. Gubbels, J. Brant, J. B. Hunter, B. Isaacson, J. Walter Kutz, R. K. Gurgel, D. M. Zeitler, C. A. Buchman, J. B. Firszt, R. H. Gifford, D. S. Haynes, R. F. Labadie, and Cochlear Implant Quality of Life Development Consortium. 2019. Cochlear Implant Quality of Life (CIQOL): Development of a profile instrument (CIQOL-35 Profile) and a global measure (CIQOL-10 Global). *Journal of Speech, Language, and Hearing Research* 62(9):3554–3563.

Meinzen-Derr, J., S. Wiley, J. Creighton, and D. Choo. 2007. Auditory skills checklist: Clinical tool for monitoring functional auditory skill development in young children with cochlear implants. *Annals of Otology, Rhinology and Laryngology* 116(11):812–818.

Mendel, L. L., W. D. Mustain, and J. Magro. 2014. Normative data for the Maryland CNC test. *Journal of the American Academy of Audiology* 25(8):775–781.

Meyer, T. A., and D. B. Pisoni. 1999. Some computational analyses of the PBK test: Effects of frequency and lexical density on spoken word recognition. *Ear and Hearing* 20(4):363–371.

Mishra, S. K., S. P. Boddupally, and D. Rayapati. 2015. Auditory learning in children with cochlear implants. *Journal of Speech, Language, and Hearing Research* 58(3):1052–1060.

MSTB (Minimum Speech Test Battery). 2011. *Minimum speech test battery for adult cochlear implant users.* http://www.auditorypotential.com/MSTBfiles/MSTBManual2011-06-20%20.pdf (accessed October 17, 2020).

Newman, C. W., B. E. Weinstein, G. P. Jacobson, and G. A. Hug. 1990. The Hearing Handicap Inventory for Adults: Psychometric adequacy and audiometric correlates. *Ear and Hearing* 11(6):430–433.

NICE (National Institute for Health and Clinical Excellence). 2019. *Cochlear implants for children and adults with severe to profound deafness.* https://www.nice.org.uk/guidance/ta566/resources/cochlear-implants-for-children-and-adults-with-severe-to-profound-deafness-pdf-82607085698245 (accessed October 15, 2020).

Nilsson, M., S. D. Soli, and J. A. Sullivan. 1994. Development of the Hearing in Noise Test for the measurement of speech reception thresholds in quiet and in noise. *Journal of the Acoustical Society of America* 95(2):1085–1099.

Nilsson, M. J., S. D. Soli, and D. J. Gelnett. 1996. Development of the Hearing in Noise Test for Children (HINT-C). Los Angeles, CA: House Ear Institute.

Peterson, G. E., and I. Lehiste. 1962. Revised CNC lists for auditory tests. *The Journal of Speech and Hearing Disorders* 27:62–70.

Plomp, R., and A. M. Mimpen. 1979. Improving the reliability of testing the speech reception threshold for sentences. *International Journal of Audiology* 18(1):43–52.

Ramkissoon, I., A. Proctor, C. R. Lansing, and R. C. Bilger. 2002. Digit speech recognition thresholds (SRT) for non-native speakers of english. *American Journal of Audiology* 11(1):23–28.

Robbins, A. M., J. J. Renshaw, and S. W. Berry. 1991. Evaluating meaningful auditory integration in profoundly hearing-impaired children. *American Journal of Otology* 12(Suppl):144–150.

Robson, H. 2001. Using a variety of signals to improve real-ear testing. *Trends in Amplification* 5(2):77–79.

Rothauser, E. H. 1969. IEEE recommended practice for speech quality measurements. *IEEE Transactions on Audio and Electroacoustics* 17(3):225–246.

Schafer, E. C. 2010. Speech perception in noise measures for children: A critical review and case studies. *Journal of Educational, Pediatric, & (Re)Habilitative Audiology* 16:4–15.

Silverman, S. R., and I. J. Hirsh. 1955. CX problems related to the use of speech in clinical audiometry. *Annals of Otology, Rhinology and Laryngology* 64(4):1234–1244.

Smits, C., and T. Houtgast. 2005. Results from the Dutch speech-in-noise screening test by telephone. *Ear and Hearing* 26(1):89–95.

Smits, C., T. S. Kapteyn, and T. Houtgast. 2004. Development and validation of an automatic speech-in-noise screening test by telephone. *International Journal of Audiology* 43(1):15–28.

Smits, C., P. Merkus, and T. Houtgast. 2006. How we do it: The Dutch functional hearing-screening tests by telephone and internet. *Clinical Otolaryngology* 31(5):436–440.

Spahr, A. J., and M. F. Dorman. 2005. Effects of minimum stimulation settings for the MED EL Tempo+ speech processor on speech understanding. *Ear and Hearing* 26(4 Suppl):2S–6S.

Spahr, A. J., M. F. Dorman, and L. H. Loiselle. 2007. Performance of patients using different cochlear implant systems: Effects of input dynamic range. *Ear and Hearing* 28(2):260–275.

Spahr, A. J., M. F. Dorman, L. M. Litvak, S. Van Wie, R. H. Gifford, P. C. Loizou, L. M. Loiselle, T. Oakes, and S. Cook. 2012. Development and validation of the AzBio sentence lists. *Ear and Hearing* 33(1):112–117.

Spahr, A. J., M. F. Dorman, L. M. Litvak, S. J. Cook, L. M. Loiselle, M. D. DeJong, A. Hedley-Williams, L. S. Sunderhaus, C. A. Hayes, and R. H. Gifford. 2014. Development and validation of the Pediatric AzBio sentence lists. *Ear and Hearing* 35(4):418–422.

Stam, M., C. Smits, J. W. Twisk, U. Lemke, J. M. Festen, and S. E. Kramer. 2015. Deterioration of speech recognition ability over a period of 5 years in adults ages 18 to 70 years: Results of the Dutch online speech-in-noise test. *Ear and Hearing* 36(3):e129–e137.

Thornton, A. R., and M. J. M. Raffin. 1978. Speech-discrimination scores modeled as a binomial variable. *Journal of Speech and Hearing Research* 21(3):507–518.

Tillman, T. W., and R. Carhart. 1966. *An expanded test for speech discrimination utilizing CNC monosyllabic words.* Northwestern University Auditory Test no. 6. Technical report SAM-TR-66-55. Brooks Air Force Base, Texas: USAF School of Aerospace Medicine. https://pdfs.semanticscholar.org/008e/54f6708d34231a350af7e7b585b53a8c048c.pdf (accessed January 15, 2021).

Tillman, T. W., R. Cahart, and W. O. Olsen. 1970. Hearing aid efficiency in a competing speech situation. *Journal of Speech and Hearing Research* 13(4):789–811.

Ventry, I. M., and B. E. Weinstein. 1982. The Hearing Handicap Inventory for the Elderly: A new tool. *Ear and Hearing* 3(3):128–134.

Wackym, P. A., C. L. Runge-Samuelson, J. B. Firszt, F. M. Alkaf, and L. S. Burg. 2007. More challenging speech-perception tasks demonstrate binaural benefit in bilateral cochlear implant users. *Ear and Hearing* 28(Suppl 2):80S–85S.

Watson, C. S., G. R. Kidd, J. D. Miller, C. Smits, and L. E. Humes. 2012. Telephone screening tests for functionally impaired hearing: Current use in seven countries and development of a U.S. version. *Journal of the American Academy of Audiology* 23(10):757–767.

Weichbold, V., L. Tsiakpini, F. Coninx, and P. D'Haese. 2005. Development of a parent questionnaire for assessment of auditory behaviour of infants up to two years of age. *Laryngo-Rhino-Otologie* 84(5):328–334.

Williams-Sanchez, V., R. A. McArdle, R. H. Wilson, G. R. Kidd, C. S. Watson, and A. L. Bourne. 2014. Validation of a screening test of auditory function using the telephone. *Journal of the American Academy of Audiology* 25(10):937–951.

Wilson, R. H., and A. Strouse. 2002. Northwestern University Auditory Test no. 6 in multi-talker babble: A preliminary report. *Journal of Rehabilitation Research and Development* 39(1):105–114.

Wilson, R. H., H. B. Abrams, and A. L. Pillion. 2003. A word-recognition task in multitalker babble using a descending presentation mode from 24 db to 0 db signal to babble. *Journal of Rehabilitation Research and Development* 40(4):321–327.

Wilson, R. H., R. A. McArdle, and S. L. Smith. 2007. An evaluation of the BKB–SIN, HINT, QuickSIN, and WIN materials on listeners with normal hearing and listeners with hearing loss. *Journal of Speech, Language, and Hearing Research* 50(4):844–856.

Zimmerman-Phillips, S., A. McConkey Robbins, and M. J. Osberger. 2000. Assessing cochlear implant benefit in very young children. *Annals of Otology, Rhinology and Laryngology* 109(12 II Suppl):42–43.

5

Evaluating Hearing Ability in Persons with Cochlear Implants with Single-Sided Deafness or Asymmetric Hearing Loss

This chapter will address item 4 from the Statement of Task, which directs the committee to:

Examine the special considerations inherent in evaluating hearing ability in persons with single-sided deafness or asymmetric hearing loss receiving a cochlear implant and to describe the following:

a. Any special considerations in the testing and treatment of persons with bilateral but unequal hearing loss;
b. Whether there is a correlation between the presence and degree of hearing loss in the less-affected ear and the recovery time or treatment for individuals with single-sided deafness or asymmetric hearing loss receiving a cochlear implant in their more-affected ear;
c. Whether there is a level of hearing ability in the less-affected ear which would render cochlear implantation in the more-affected ear immaterial with respect to meeting the severity of hearing loss in the Listings (i.e., would not prevent an adult from engaging in any gainful activity nor a child from having "marked" limitations in two domains of functioning or an "extreme" limitation in one domain[1]);
d. Whether the tests identified in task 3 remain appropriate for testing hearing ability in persons with single-sided deafness or asymmetric

---

[1] See 20 Code of Federal Regulations 416.926a and DI (disability insurance) 25225.030, DI 25225.035, DI 25225.040, DI 25225.045, DI 25225.050, and DI 25225.055.

hearing loss receiving a cochlear implant and why, and if there are any differences in how the tests should be administered or interpreted; and

e. Whether the equivalent scores identified in task 3 remain accurate proxies for the HINT word recognition scores when assessing persons with single-sided deafness or asymmetric hearing loss receiving a cochlear implant.

The chapter begins with background information and challenges for the U.S. Social Security Administration (SSA) in regard to single-sided deafness (SSD) and asymmetric hearing loss (AHL) in individuals with cochlear implants. The chapter also provides an overview of special considerations inherent in evaluating hearing ability in patients with SSD or AHL who receive a cochlear implant. Finally, the committee responds to each of the items, in the order in which they appear, in the Statement of Task.

INTRODUCTION

Hearing loss can be classified as bilateral hearing loss, unilateral hearing loss (UHL), or AHL on the basis of its lateral differentiation and degree of severity. Bilateral hearing loss is a general term for hearing loss in both ears, regardless of severity. UHL is a general term for hearing loss in only one ear, regardless of severity. AHL is defined as hearing loss in both ears, with a difference in pure tone averages (PTAs)[2] between the two ears. The exact criteria for difference in PTA varies in the literature (Liu et al., 2020). SSD is UHL in which hearing loss in the impaired ear is severe to profound, most often caused by sudden sensorineural hearing loss (Giardina et al., 2014). There is some disagreement in the literature on the specific definition of SSD, and some authors categorize some forms of SSD as a type of AHL rather than UHL (Liu et al., 2020). With regard to cochlear implantation, the U.S. Food and Drug Administration (FDA) currently defines AHL as a profound sensorineural hearing loss in one ear and mild to moderately severe sensorineural hearing loss in the other ear, with a difference of at least 15 decibels (dB) in PTAs between ears (FDA, 2020). It defines SSD as a profound sensorineural hearing loss in one ear and normal hearing or mild sensorineural hearing loss in the other ear (FDA, 2020).

The prevalence of UHL in adult Americans has been estimated to be 7.2 percent, with 1.5 percent experiencing moderate or severe UHL (i.e., SSD) (Golub et al., 2018). The prevalence of UHL in children has been estimated at approximately 1 congenital UHL per 1,000 births, increasing

---

[2] The average of hearing threshold levels at a set of specified frequencies (e.g., 0.5, 1, 2, and 4 kHz).

to an estimated 14 percent when one includes delayed-onset congenital UHL and acquired etiologies among adolescents ages 12–19 years (Lieu, 2018). Hassepass et al. (2013) estimated an SSD prevalence of 2–5 percent in children and teenagers. A recent study estimated AHL prevalence in the United States using data from the National Health and Nutrition Examination Survey and two definitions of AHL (Suen et al., 2021). Using the American Academy of Otolaryngology—Head and Neck Surgery definition of AHL as a PTA difference of greater than 15 dB, the researchers found an overall AHL prevalence of 2.77 and 9.46 percent when calculating the PTA with 0.5–4 kHz and 4–8 kHz, respectively. In contrast, using the U.S. Department of Veterans Affairs definition of AHL as a difference greater than/equal to 20 dB across two contiguous frequencies or 10 dB across three contiguous frequencies, the authors calculated an overall prevalence of 25.05 percent across 0.5–8 kHz (Suen et al., 2021).

The committee notes that when cochlear implants were first approved, they were intended for use with adults and children with bilateral profound sensorineural hearing loss. Over the years, the safety and efficacy of cochlear implants have been well established, and their approval for use has been expanded to include patients with greater amounts of hearing. FDA approved cochlear implants for use in patients with SSD and AHL (FDA, 2019a). As a result, many insurers now cover the cost of cochlear implants for patients with SSD and AHL and will consider approving cochlear implants for patients who do not meet FDA-approved indications but who have been determined by a medical professional to be suitable to receive a device (a practice referred to as "off-label use" of a medical device) (FDA, 2020).

Those changes in practice regarding who receives a cochlear implant pose special challenges for SSA for several reasons. First, current indications for disability due to hearing loss not treated with cochlear implantation (SSA Listing 2.10) base eligibility on the hearing in the better hearing ear; individuals will qualify for disability if they have an average air conduction hearing threshold of 90 dB or greater in the better ear and an average bone conduction hearing threshold of 60 dB or greater in the better ear (2.00B2c) or if they have a word recognition score of 40 percent correct or less in the better ear determined using a standardized list of phonetically balanced monosyllabic words (2.00B2e). Presently, SSA considers an individual who receives a cochlear implant to be under a disability for 1 year after initial implantation or, if more than 1 year after implantation, a word recognition score of 60 percent correct or less determined using the Hearing in Noise Test (HINT) (2.00B2b). It is evident that those guidelines were based on the underlying assumption that cochlear implants were primarily being used by individuals who demonstrated a significant and impactful bilateral sensorineural hearing loss. However, that is no longer the case.

The presence of normal or near-normal hearing in one ear, which is the case for individuals with SSD or AHL who receive a cochlear implant, has complicated the determination of disability due to hearing loss. Historically, professionals have assumed that the presence of normal hearing in one ear provides sufficient auditory input to result in a relatively normal hearing experience (Giardina et al., 2014). Thus, SSD and AHL often went untreated. Recent research has identified several difficulties that patients with UHL or AHL face, including difficulty hearing in complex or noisy environments and an inability to identify the location or laterality of sounds (Kamal et al., 2012) as well as an increased prevalence of tinnitus (Liu et al., 2018). The presence of SSD or AHL can be particularly impactful for children and has been found to result in delays in auditory behavior (Kishon-Rabin et al., 2015); reduced communication, motor skills, and adaptive behavior (Vohr et al., 2012); delays in the development of speech and language (Fischer and Lieu, 2014; Lieu et al., 2013; Sangen et al., 2017); a higher incidence of behavior issues (Lieu et al., 2012); and a reduction in self-reported quality of life (Rachakonda et al., 2014; Umansky et al., 2011). Because these difficulties have been noted, professionals are now more likely to recommend intervention for SSD and AHL in both children and adults than in the past.

The safety and efficacy of treating SSD and AHL with a cochlear implant has been demonstrated in both children and adults (FDA, 2019b). However, due to changes regarding who is considered to be a candidate for a cochlear implant, it is necessary to re-examine the disability coverage related to cochlear implantation. It needs to be determined whether patients with SSD and AHL who receive a cochlear implant and possess normal or near-normal hearing in one ear should automatically be covered under disability for a period of 1 year after they receive the cochlear implant.

SPECIAL CONSIDERATION IN THE TESTING AND TREATMENT OF PERSONS WITH BILATERAL BUT UNEQUAL HEARING LOSS

Hearing Testing

Hearing can be measured unilaterally (one ear at a time), bilaterally (each ear separately), or binaurally (both ears tested together at the same time). Additionally, hearing testing can be performed in either an unaided or aided condition. Unaided testing provides a measure of hearing sensitivity without the use of hearing technology and is typically performed using insert earphones and a bone conduction oscillator. The results of such testing provide information regarding the type and severity of the hearing loss. When testing is done in an aided condition, the patient uses hearing assistance, such as a hearing aid or cochlear implant. For patients who use hearing technology, this testing is often used to investigate the patient's typical hearing situation, and a comparison of unaided and aided responses can be used to estimate the amount of benefit a patient will receive from the hearing technology.

When hearing testing reveals the presence of hearing loss, the loss can be unilateral (present in only one ear) or bilateral (present in both ears). In unilateral hearing loss, the severity of the hearing loss in the affected ear can range from mild to profound while the non-affected ear typically has normal hearing.

There are special considerations that need to be addressed when testing the hearing of individuals with unequal hearing in the two ears. During testing the examiner needs to ensure that steps are taken to control for the possibility that sound presented to one ear (the test ear) may cross over and be heard by the other (non-test) ear. Such steps should be applied to signals delivered via air conduction, via bone conduction, and during speech recognition testing, and they should be taken during both unaided and aided testing.

Unaided Testing

During unaided testing, masking noise is typically delivered to the non-test ear via insert earphones, and the level of masking is determined by several factors, including the air and bone conduction thresholds of the non-test ear, the air conduction threshold of the test ear, and the level of presentation of the signal in the test ear. The masking level is also influenced by such factors as interaural attenuation (IA), a reduction in intensity of the stimulus as sound is transmitted from one ear to the other across the listener's head. IA will vary depending on the equipment used to deliver the stimulus and is typically estimated to be a minimum of 40 dB for supra-aural headphones, 50 dB for insert earphones, and 0 dB for bone conduction. When presenting a masking stimulus, the examiner must be careful not to provide too much masking noise to the non-test ear as doing so may cause the masking noise to cross over to the test ear and affect the results (overmasking).

Aided Testing

It is also important to control for possible perception of the test signal by the non-test ear when testing patients with unequal hearing in an aided condition. Typically, the purpose of such testing is to determine the efficacy of the intervention and the benefit it provides when tested alone, without the influence of the other ear, and to determine the benefit that use of the technology provides when tested in a binaural listening condition (which more likely represents the patient's everyday listening situation). Techniques that can be used during aided testing to isolate the affected ear and block perception of the signal by the non-test ear include removal of the hearing aid or cochlear implant from the non-test ear, plugging of the non-test ear, plugging and muffling of the non-test ear, the delivery of masking noise to the non-test ear, and the use of direct connection to the hearing technology of the test ear. Those techniques may be used in isolation or in combination with one another depending on the amount of hearing present in the non-test and test ears and the level of signal being presented to the test ear. The above-mentioned signal control methods are typically used when evaluating speech understanding in quiet or in noise. Other measures used to evaluate the efficacy of devices include questionnaires that examine quality of life and tinnitus (Van de Heyning et al., 2017).

Treatment Options

Treatment options for patients with UHL and AHL are determined by the type and severity of the loss in the affected ear. Patients with mild to severe UHL (i.e., SSD) may choose to use a hearing aid in the affected ear or may choose to deny or defer treatment of the affected ear. The affected ear is often left untreated as some believe that the presence of normal hearing in at least one ear is sufficient for daily hearing function. Recent research, however, has shed additional light on this topic, and currently most professionals believe that treatment of mild to severe UHL (i.e., SSD) is warranted. The ability to successfully treat hearing loss in the affected ear will depend on the type and severity of the hearing loss as well as on the speech recognition skills of the affected ear. Additionally, a decision to treat an ear may be affected by other factors, such as the presence of tinnitus or balance issues in the affected ear. Possible treatment options for UHL include hearing aids (either air conduction or bone conduction), surgical treatment in the case of conductive or mixed losses, or the surgical insertion of a cochlear implant.

Because of the significant nature of the hearing loss in the affected ear, patients with SSD or AHL pose special treatment challenges because the affected ear typically cannot receive benefit from traditional technologies, such as an air conduction hearing aid. Thus, treatment options for such patients include use of devices that pick up sound on the side of the affected ear and transmit it to the ear with normal hearing, such as a Contralateral Routing of Signal (CROS) hearing aid. CROS aids place a microphone on the affected ear that picks up sound and transmits it to the ear with normal hearing via an air-conducted signal. In cases of AHL, if an aidable loss is present in the better-hearing ear, the patient may be fit with a bilateral CROS. This is similar to a CROS, but the hearing aid used to provide sound to the better hearing ear is amplified. Alternatively, the surgical or non-surgical placement of a bone conduction device can be used to provide sound awareness on the side of the head with the hearing loss. Like the CROS, bone conduction devices pick up sound on the side of the affected ear and transmit it to the ear with normal hearing. However, the transmission of the signal is done via use of a bone-conducted, rather than an air-conducted, signal. Because these devices route the signal from both sides of the head to the ear with normal hearing, they are not considered binaural solutions.

The only treatment option that provides truly binaural hearing for SSD patients or patients with an AHL with an ear that has profound hearing loss is a cochlear implant. As has been explained previously, cochlear implants include surgical placement of an electrode array into the cochlea of the affected ear, with the patient using an externally worn sound processor that picks up sound from the environment and sends the signal to the implanted electrode array, which stimulates the inner ear and provides sound information to the brain. Cochlear implants received FDA approval for use in patients aged 5 years and older with AHL or SSD in 2018 (FDA, 2019a).

It should be noted that patients with SSD often experience tinnitus in the affected ear. In some instances the tinnitus is debilitating. Because cochlear implants frequently help reduce tinnitus (Arts et al., 2012; Servais et al., 2017), the presence of severe tinnitus in the affected ear may provide additional support for a recommendation for a cochlear implant. Many insurers recognize the value of hearing from both ears and provide coverage for both bone conduction devices and cochlear implants as treatments for SSD.

CORRELATION BETWEEN HEARING LOSS IN THE LESS-AFFECTED EAR AND RECOVERY TIME OR TREATMENT IN THE MORE-AFFECTED EAR

This section discusses whether there is a correlation between the presence and degree of hearing loss in the less-affected ear and the recovery time or treatment of individuals with SSD or AHL receiving a cochlear implant in their more-affected ear.

Surgery and Recovery Time

Cochlear implantation involves the surgical placement of an electrode array into the cochlea. Typically, cochlear implant surgery lasts about 2–3 hours and is performed under general anesthesia. A few investigators have reported success performing cochlear implant surgeries under local anesthesia and sedation (Connors et al., 2021). The recovery time following surgery can be influenced by several factors, including the patient's reaction to anesthesia, the need for medication for pain reduction, and swelling at the incision site. In most instances, adults and children return to their normal routine when they feel well enough to do so, often within a few days of surgery. Patients are typically seen by their surgeon either in the clinic or virtually via telemedicine for an inspection of the incision about 1 week following surgery. In most clinics, the external device is activated 2–4 weeks after surgery and in some cases has been reported as early as 1 day following surgery (Hagr et al., 2015).

Activating a cochlear implant involves several different steps, including impedance telemetry, setting the levels of the electrodes, adjusting the levels when the patient is exposed to live speech, and downloading of the programs to the sound processor. Patients are typically provided with successively louder programs to use over the coming few weeks as they adjust to the overall loudness of the electric signal. In most clinics adults return 1, 3, 6, and 12 months post-activation for follow-up (Dunn, 2018), while children return slightly more often. During these appointments, the clinician reassesses the levels of the electrodes, reviews device use and care with the patient and his or her parent(s), and evaluates performance with the device.

How well an individual adjusts to the sound quality of the device varies greatly among those who receive a cochlear implant. Adjustment can be difficult for some patients, and that may affect both their device use and the amount of benefit they receive from the device. Children frequently participate in weekly therapy provided by a speech–language pathologist that helps them learn to use the speech information provided by the cochlear implant. Adults also might participate in such therapy, but recommendations for such therapy are less prevalent in the adult population.

When adults and children (ages 5 years and older) with SSD or AHL receive a cochlear implant, they typically participate in the same number and type of post-operative appointments as traditional cochlear implant recipients. The adjustment to sound quality and ability to recognize speech with the device is similar to the adjustment that takes place with traditional recipients and will vary among individuals. The presence of reduced speech recognition in the implanted ear soon after receiving a cochlear implant is somewhat common. However, reduced speech recognition with the cochlear implant is not as detrimental or as difficult for adult or pediatric patients with SSD or AHL as they are able to rely on the hearing ability of their normal hearing or near-normal hearing ear to communicate. The presence of good hearing in at least one ear will likely prevent an adult from meeting the indication of "being unable to engage in any gainful activity" and will likely also prevent a child from meeting the indication of "having marked limitations in two domains of functioning or an extreme limitation in one domain."

SINGLE-SIDED DEAFNESS, ASYMMETRIC HEARING LOSS, AND SOCIAL SECURITY DISABILITY

This section will discuss whether there is a level of hearing ability in the less-affected ear that would render cochlear implantation in the more-affected ear immaterial with respect to meeting the severity of hearing loss in the *Listing of Impairments* (the Listings) (i.e., would not prevent an adult from engaging in any gainful activity nor a child from having "marked" limitations in two domains of functioning or an "extreme" limitation in one domain).

Historically, indications to qualify for a cochlear implant and indications to qualify for disability due to hearing loss have required patients to have a significant *bilateral* hearing loss. With cochlear implants, this was a decision made in early clinical trials when the safety and efficacy of cochlear implants were not yet proven. The decision to provide cochlear implants to patients with significant SSD or AHL was made only recently, when FDA approved cochlear implants for adults and children (ages 5 and up) with SSD and AHL (FDA, 2019a). This decision was based on research demonstrating that most individuals with SSD or AHL demonstrated improvements in word and sentence recognition in quiet in the implanted ear, improvements in sentence recognition in noise when noise was presented to the better hearing ear, improvements in sound localization, and improvements in self-perceived quality of hearing (FDA, 2019b).

The presence of a bilateral profound hearing loss not treated with a cochlear implant will likely prevent adults from engaging in any gainful activity and will likely result in children having marked limitations in various domains of functioning. Currently, patients without a cochlear implant qualify for Listings-level disability if they demonstrate an average air conduction hearing threshold of 90 dB or greater in the better ear and an average bone conduction hearing threshold of 60 dB or greater in the better ear (2.10A) or if they demonstrate a word recognition score of 40 percent correct or less in the better ear determined using a standardized list of phonetically balanced monosyllabic words (2.10B). Thus, patients' hearing loss must be bilateral and must have a significant impact on their ability to communicate. If an adult patient's hearing loss has been treated with a cochlear implant, he or she is considered under disability for 1 year after initial implantation (2.11A). On occasion, adults and children will continue to demonstrate difficulty hearing even after receiving a cochlear implant. When this occurs, the individual can still qualify for disability by scoring 60 percent correct or less on word recognition using the HINT Sentences test (2.11B, 102.11).

Most adults and children with bilateral significant hearing loss who receive a cochlear implant derive benefit from the device, and the improvements they receive often prevent them from qualifying for disability after 1 year of using the device. Buchman et al. (2020) recently reported post-operative sentence recognition scores for 96 adults with bilateral moderate to profound sensorineural hearing losses who received a cochlear implant and participated in a multicenter prospective clinical trial. The subjects demonstrated mean preoperative word scores of 14.6 and 28.8 percent for the implant ear and in a bimodal test condition, respectively. Six months post-implant the mean scores improved to 60.9 percent in the implant ear (range = 56.6 to 65.2) and 69.2 percent in the bimodal condition, meaning cochlear implant in one ear and hearing aid in the other ear (range = 65.4 to 73.1). Test stimuli were presented in quiet at a level of 60 dB SPL, which is softer (and more difficult) than the 60 dB HL presentation level currently used to determine disability under current SSA requirements. Thus, most of these patients would not have qualified for continuing disability under current SSA indications.

As indicated previously, cochlear implants were not yet approved by FDA for use in patients with SSD or AHL when the current SSA guidelines were developed. Prior to the approval of cochlear implants for SSD and AHL, indications for cochlear implants, like indications for disability, were based on the "best" hearing situation. Thus, most cochlear implant recipients who were implanted previously qualified for disability under both 2.10 and 2.11 prior to receiving a cochlear implant since they likely experienced significant hearing loss in each ear. *This would not be the case for patients who currently receive a cochlear implant due to SSD or AHL because they possess normal or near-normal hearing in their better ear.*

Under current SSA guidelines, patients with SSD or AHL automatically qualify for disability for a period of 1 year following cochlear implantation, with no consideration given to the hearing in their better ear. To remain consistent with the wording and rationale used in current guidelines for hearing loss not treated with cochlear implantation (2.10 and 102.10), it is reasonable to consider the hearing in the better ear when determining whether a patient with a cochlear implant qualifies for disability due to hearing loss after they receive a cochlear implant.

TESTING HEARING ABILITY IN PERSONS WITH SINGLE-SIDED DEAFNESS OR ASYMMETRIC HEARING LOSS RECEIVING A COCHLEAR IMPLANT

SSA asked the committee whether the tests identified in task 3 of the Statement of Task remain appropriate for testing hearing ability in persons with SSD or AHL receiving a cochlear implant and why and also if there are any differences in how the tests should be administered or interpreted. The committee finds that the same tests and testing parameters can be used, with a few additional considerations. Testing for disability for hearing loss has typically focused on the test results obtained with the better ear. Thus, a patient who receives a cochlear implant due to SSD or AHL should be required to participate in testing that represents the listening situation that they use on a daily basis, which typically includes an un-occluded better ear and an ear using hearing technology. Alternatively, testing could be based on the individual being required to meet current requirements for hearing loss not treated with cochlear implantation in the ear that does not contain the device (2.10).

PROXIES FOR THE HEARING IN NOISE TEST FOR INDIVIDUALS WITH SINGLE-SIDED DEAFNESS OR ASYMMETRIC HEARING LOSS

The committee was asked to determine whether the equivalent scores identified in task 3 remain accurate proxies for the HINT word recognition scores when assessing persons with SSD or AHL receiving a cochlear implant. As indicated in Chapter 4, an accurate proxy for the HINT word recognition test does not currently exist. It should be noted, however, that the measures that will be proposed in Chapter 6 to determine disability for hearing loss treated with cochlear implants are applicable to individuals with SSD and AHL. Because such individuals typically use the cochlear implant in conjunction with the hearing in their normal or near-normal nonimplanted ear, testing should be performed while the individual uses the hearing in both ears (Sladen et al., 2017).

REFERENCES

Arts, R. A. G. J., E. L. J. George, R. J. Stokroos, and K. Vermeire. 2012. Review: Cochlear implants as a treatment of tinnitus in single-sided deafness. *Current Opinion in Otolaryngology and Head and Neck Surgery* 20(5):398–403.

Buchman, C. A., J. A. Herzog, J. L. McJunkin, C. C. Wick, N. Durakovic, J. B. Firszt, D. Kallogjeri, C. A. Buchman, J. A. Herzog, J. L. McJunkin, C. C. Wick, N. Durakovic, J. B. Firszt, D. Kallogjeri, A. Drescher, L. Holden, N. Dwyer, L. Beyer, S. Rathgeb, L. Potts, K. Mispagel, B. Peters, Y. Hahn, K. King, L. Lianos, B. Perry, S. King, J. Evans, L. Luduena, M. Wood, S. Baker, M. Duke, S. Neumann, J. Wolfe, R. Cullen, J. Ursick, K. Lewis, S. Zlmoke, M. Nelson, S. Waltzman, T. Roland, D. Jethanamest, D. Friedman, L. Mahoney, A. Rigby, B. Shapiro, O. F. Adunka, A. Moberly, E. Dodson, K. Vasil, D. Kelsall, E. Lupo, A. Biever, N. Giddings, J. Ziegler, P. Polennsky-Boner, C. Limb, A. Tward, K. Kramer, B. Gantz, M. Hansen, C. Dunn, J. Beecher, T. van Voorst, S. Karsten, T. Zwolan, H. El-Kashlan, S. Telian, H. Slager, and C. I. S. Group. 2020. Assessment of speech understanding after cochlear implantation in adult hearing aid users a nonrandomized controlled trial. *JAMA Otolaryngology—Head and Neck Surgery* 146(10):916–924.

Connors, J. R., N. L. Deep, T. K. Huncke, and J. T. Roland, Jr. 2021. Cochlear implantation under local anesthesia with conscious sedation in the elderly: First 100 cases. *Laryngoscope* 131(3):E946–E951.

Dunn, C. 2018. *Word recognition and audiometric profiles of cochlear implant candidacy.* Paper read at Emerging Issues in Cochlear Implantation CI2018 Meeting, Washington, DC. https://www.acialliance.org/page/CI2018 (accessed September 24, 2020).

FDA (U.S. Food and Drug Administration). 2019a. *MED-EL cochlear implant system—P000025/S104.* https://www.fda.gov/medical-devices/recently-approved-devices/med-el-cochlear-implant-system-p000025s104 (accessed September 24, 2020).

FDA. 2019b. *Summary of safety and effectiveness data (SSED).* https://www.accessdata.fda.gov/cdrh_docs/pdf/P000025S104B.pdf (accessed September 24, 2020).

FDA. 2020. *"Off-label" and investigational use of marketed drugs, biologics, and medical devices.* https://www.fda.gov/regulatory-information/search-fda-guidance-documents/label-and-investigational-use-marketed-drugs-biologics-and-medical-devices (accessed September 24, 2020).

Fischer, C., and J. Lieu. 2014. Unilateral hearing loss is associated with a negative effect on language scores in adolescents. *International Journal of Pediatric Otorhinolaryngology* 78(10):1611–1617.

Giardina, C. K., E. J. Formeister, and O. F. Adunka. 2014. Cochlear implants in single-sided deafness. *Current Surgery Reports* 2(12):75.

Golub, J. S., F. R. Lin, L. R. Lustig, and A. K. Lalwani. 2018. Prevalence of adult unilateral hearing loss and hearing aid use in the United States. *Laryngoscope* 128(7):1681–1686.

Hagr, A., S. N. Garadat, M. Al-Momani, R. M. Alsabellha, and F. A. Almuhawas. 2015. Feasibility of one-day activation in cochlear implant recipients. *International Journal of Audiology* 54(5):323–328.

Hassepass, F., A. Aschendorff, T. Wesarg, S. Kröger, R. Laszig, R. L. Beck, C. Schild, and S. Arndt. 2013. Unilateral deafness in children: Audiologic and subjective assessment of hearing ability after cochlear implantation. *Otology and Neurotology* 34(1):53–60.

Kamal, S. M., A. D. Robinson, and R. C. Diaz. 2012. Cochlear implantation in single-sided deafness for enhancement of sound localization and speech perception. *Current Opinion in Otolaryngology and Head and Neck Surgery* 20(5):393–397.

Kishon-Rabin, L., J. Kuint, M. Hildesheimer, and D. Ari-Even Roth. 2015. Delay in auditory behaviour and preverbal vocalization in infants with unilateral hearing loss. *Developmental Medicine and Child Neurology* 57(12):1129–1136.

Lieu, J. E. C. 2018. Permanent unilateral hearing loss (UHL) and childhood development. *Current Otorhinolaryngology Reports* 6(1):74–81.

Lieu, J. E. C., N. Tye-Murray, and Q. Fu. 2012. Longitudinal study of children with unilateral hearing loss. *Laryngoscope* 122(9):2088–2095.

Lieu, J. E. C., R. K. Karzon, B. Ead, and N. Tye-Murray. 2013. Do audiologic characteristics predict outcomes in children with unilateral hearing loss? *Otology and Neurotology* 34(9):1703–1710.

Liu, Y. W., X. Cheng, B. Chen, K. Peng, A. Ishiyama, and Q. J. Fu. 2018. Effect of tinnitus and duration of deafness on sound localization and speech recognition in noise in patients with single-sided deafness. *Trends in Hearing* 22:2331216518813802.

Liu, J., M. Zhou, X. He, and N. Wang. 2020. Single-sided deafness and unilateral auditory deprivation in children: Current challenge of improving sound localization ability. *Journal of International Medical Research* 48(1):300060519896912.

Rachakonda, T., D. B. Jeffe, J. J. Shin, L. Mankarious, R. J. Fanning, M. M. Lesperance, and J. E. C. Lieu. 2014. Validity, discriminative ability, and reliability of the hearing-related quality of life questionnaire for adolescents. *Laryngoscope* 124(2):570–578.

Sangen, A., L. Royackers, C. Desloovere, J. Wouters, and A. van Wieringen. 2017. Single-sided deafness affects language and auditory development—A case–control study. *Clinical Otolaryngology* 42(5):979–987.

Servais, J. J., K. Hörmann, and E. Wallhäusser-Franke. 2017. Unilateral cochlear implantation reduces tinnitus loudness in bimodal hearing: A prospective study. *Frontiers in Neurology* 8:60.
Sladen, D. P., R. H. Gifford, D. Haynes, D. Kelsall, A. Benson, K. Lewis, T. Zwolan, Q. J. Fu, B. Gantz, J. Gilden, B. Westerberg, C. Gustin, L. O'Neil, and C. L. Driscoll. 2017. Evaluation of a revised indication for determining adult cochlear implant candidacy. *Laryngoscope* 127(10):2368–2374.
Suen, J. J., J. Betz, N. S. Reed, J. A. Deal, F. R. Lin, and A. M. Goman. 2021. Prevalence of asymmetric hearing among adults in the United States. *Otology & Neurotology* 42(2):e111–e113.
Umansky, A. M., D. B. Jeffe, and J. E. C. Lieu. 2011. The HEAR-QL: Quality of life questionnaire for children with hearing loss. *Journal of the American Academy of Audiology* 22(10):644–653.
Van De Heyning, P., D. Távora-Vieira, G. Mertens, V. Van Rompaey, G. P. Rajan, J. Müller, J. M. Hempel, D. Leander, D. Polterauer, M. Marx, S. I. Usami, R. Kitoh, M. Miyagawa, H. Moteki, K. Smilsky, W. D. Baumgartner, T. G. Keintzel, G. M. Sprinzl, A. Wolf-Magele, S. Arndt, T. Wesarg, S. Zirn, U. Baumann, T. Weissgerber, T. Rader, R. Hagen, A. Kurz, K. Rak, R. Stokroos, E. George, R. Polo, M. D. M. Medina, Y. Henkin, O. Hilly, D. Ulanovski, R. Rajeswaran, M. Kameswaran, M. F. Di Gregorio, and M. E. Zernotti. 2017. Towards a unified testing framework for single-sided deafness studies: A consensus paper. *Audiology and Neurotology* 21(6):391–398.
Vohr, B., D. Topol, N. Girard, L. St. Pierre, V. Watson, and R. Tucker. 2012. Language outcomes and service provision of preschool children with congenital hearing loss. *Early Human Development* 88(7):493–498.

6

Test Comparisons and Recommendations

This chapter addresses the third item in the Statement of Task:

Among the hearing tests discussed in task 2 of the Statement of Task, identify those with characteristics most similar to the Hearing in Noise Test (HINT), determine which tests, performed in the sound field, either binaurally or monaurally, in either quiet or noise, produce measurements most closely analogous to the word recognition score of the HINT (given HINT testing parameters of properly functioning cochlear implants set at normal settings, with no visual testing cues, in a quiet sound field, at 60 dB HL), and describe to the degree possible:

a. What differences exist between the identified tests and the HINT in terms of the specific elements of hearing ability they measure;
b. The committee's recommendations as to how scores from the identified tests can be compared or converted to equivalent scores on the HINT; and
c. The committee's recommendations for the scores on hearing tests that correspond to a level of functional hearing ability that causes marked and severe functional limitation; whether those scores or outcome measures can be expressed in a form comparable between hearing tests such as percentile or standard deviation from the norm.

Nearly 50 years ago, speech in noise measurement was recommended by Carhart and Tillman (1970) as an ecologically valid measure of communication. Since then, speech-in-noise measures have become the norm for several aspects of audiologic evaluation including the assessment of cochlear implantation. However, there remains a paucity of speech-in-noise assessments and accompanying information on the validity and reliability of materials and comparisons across materials. Given that complete information is lacking, the committee will address the third task in the Statement of Task to the degree possible, and the committee will use its expertise and judgment to make its recommendations to the U.S. Social Security Administration (SSA).

There are relatively few speech-in-noise assessments in the literature. Some of the most common sentence-in-noise tests are the HINT (Nilsson et al., 1994), the Quick Speech-in-Noise Test (QuickSIN; Killion et al., 2004), and the Bamford-Kowal-Bench Speech-in-Noise Test (BKB-SIN; Etymōtic Research, 2005; Niquette et al., 2003). Chapter 4 provides a discussion of each of those tests.

TEST COMPARISONS

McArdle et al. (2005) compared speech tests that use digits (the digit triplet test), words (the Words in Noise test, also known as the WIN), and sentences (the QuickSIN) and found the same separation of about 8 decibels (dB) between mean recognition performances by listeners with normal hearing and those with hearing loss across tests. Additionally, the authors found that the QuickSIN and the WIN produced recognition performances by listeners with hearing loss that were equivalent (about 12 dB signal-to-noise ratio [SNR]). The data from the McArdle and colleagues study suggest that the WIN and the QuickSIN provide comparable speech recognition performance in terms of the 50 percent point.

The HINT employs a different procedure to measure the 50 percent point, using an adaptive protocol in which the 50 percent point is measured by averaging the peaks and valleys of the individual psychometric tracks. Psychometric tracks refer to the data as plotted with the level of the signal on the y-axis and the presentation number on the x-axis (Wilson et al., 2007). The HINT is also scored by averaging all data points from the 4th through the 11th data point. Furthermore, the HINT uses noise that mimics the speech spectrum, whereas the other speech tests in noise use babble as background noise (Wilson et al., 2007). More normative data exist for speech recognition test materials used in quiet than for speech recognition testing in noise (Wilson et al., 2007).

Wilson et al. (2007) concluded that for both listeners with normal hearing and listeners with hearing loss, better performance was obtained on the BKB-SIN and HINT materials than on the QuickSIN and the WIN materials, although the QuickSIN and the WIN materials provided more separation in terms of a difference in performance between listeners with normal hearing and listeners with hearing loss. Wilson et al. (2007) recommend QuickSIN as the sentence test of choice and WIN for monosyllable tests. They also note that because BKB-SIN and HINT materials are easier, they should be used for protocols with young children and for individuals with severe hearing loss, such as cochlear implant candidates.

Cullington and Aidi (2017) evaluated the digit triplet test as a way to assess speech in adults with cochlear implants. They note that although sentence tests in quiet have high face validity, they may not be appropriate for all people for the following reasons:

- They can be more a test of an individual's ability to parse out context cues in a sentence;
- Language barriers can be a problem, resulting in people obtaining floor scores; and
- Performance with a cochlear implant has improved over the years, resulting in 49–71 percent of those taking the test approaching or at the ceiling on sentence testing in quiet (Firszt et al., 2004; Gifford et al., 2008), with 28 percent scoring 100 percent (Gifford et al., 2008). Near-ceiling scores can be achieved by adults with postlingual deafness after as little as 3 months of implant use (Litovsky et al., 2006). Ceiling scores are a challenge because improvements in performance over time or differences between two conditions cannot be evaluated.

A recent survey of cochlear implant clinical practice found that 100 percent of responding clinics used AzBio sentences testing and 68 percent used speech-in-noise testing to determine cochlear implant candidacy. There were no consistent SNRs[1] used for the assessment; 26 percent of clinics reported using +10 dB, 16 percent used +5 dB, and the remaining 55 percent reported using some combination of +5 and +10 dB SNR (Carlson et al., 2017).

Holder et al. (2018) tested 81 adults with normal hearing and cognitive function in a cochlear implant program, stratified by age (20–49, 50–59, 60–69, and 70–79 years). The study's purpose was to characterize speech recognition in noise for adults with normal hearing and cognitive function across the four age groups for the Arizona Biomedical (AzBio) Sentences Test, BKB-SIN, and QuickSIN. The authors hypothesized that many clinicians who are evaluating older adults for cochlear implantation prefer to not use the speech-in-noise testing for that evaluation because they believe

---

[1] The signal-to-noise ratio compares the level of a desired signal to the level of background noise.

that even older adults with normal hearing do not score well, so a poor score on that test for older adults does not necessarily indicate the need for cochlear implantation. One purpose of their study was to test that theory. Subjects completed AzBio Sentences Tests in quiet and in five SNRs (+10, +5, 0, –5, and –10 dB), as well as BKB-SIN and QuickSIN tasks. The study yielded four main findings:

1. Older adults with normal hearing exhibited ceiling-level performance for AzBio sentence recognition for all SNRs tested except for –5 and –10 dB SNR;
2. BKB-SIN data obtained in the sound field at 60 A-weighted dB (dB A) are in agreement with previously published insert earphone norms, but only for the youngest age group; all older age groups (50+ years) performed more than one standard deviation outside the published insert earphone normative data;
3. QuickSIN data obtained in the sound field were not significantly different for 60 and 70 dB A presentation levels, and the study's data replicated previously published normative data for this task; and
4. There was a significant effect of age on performance for all tests.

Based on the premise that ceiling effects are more common in the HINT than in AzBio in adults with cochlear implants, Massa and Ruckenstein (2014) conducted a retrospective review to compare 130 cochlear implant users assessed with the HINT against 125 cochlear implants users assessed with AzBio. Their results did not support the hypothesis that HINT testing would reach a performance plateau sooner. The authors found that 34 devices reached a plateau on the HINT and 30 devices reached a plateau on AzBio. Patients reached a plateau in hearing performance at similar median times using AzBio and the HINT (18.8 weeks post-operatively for the HINT, and 16.5 weeks post-operatively with AzBio) (Massa and Ruckenstein, 2014).

ALTERNATIVE MEASURES FOR THE HEARING IN NOISE TEST EQUIVALENCE

Given the historical use of the HINT sentences for measuring cochlear implant candidacy, post-operative outcomes, and SSA disability determination, it is reasonable to ask which speech recognition measures and conversion factors might be equivalent to the HINT. However, to identify validated speech recognition measures and associated conversion for HINT equivalence, one would require within- and between-subjects comparison data on a number of speech recognition measures for hundreds if not thousands of listeners. Those studies would need to demonstrate a direct comparison between HINT sentence recognition in quiet and speech recognition performance on other measures for large sample sizes in a prospective manner. Unfortunately, a body of literature meeting those criteria does not currently exist. The committee did identify one retrospective review that can inform the question, although it does not meet the aforementioned criteria required to generate a conversion value for the HINT. Gifford et al. (2008) reported speech recognition performance for 206 adult listeners with cochlear implants (n = 156) or hearing aids (n = 50) on a number of measures, including HINT sentences in quiet, consonant–nucleus–consonant (CNC) monosyllables, AzBio sentences in quiet, and BKB-SIN. When individual speech recognition performance was considered for each measure independently, the skewness of the data—an estimate of distribution asymmetry—was –1.44 for HINT sentence scores, an estimate that was more than double the skewness for all other measures tested. That is a direct result of the large proportion of listeners (28 percent) who achieved a perfect score for HINT sentences recognition in quiet as compared with the other three measures, for which < 1 percent achieved ceiling-level performance (Gifford et al., 2008).

The authors also reported the relationship between HINT sentence scores in quiet and CNC word recognition (n = 135) and BKB-SIN (n = 169) using a within-subjects, repeated-measures design. They reported that while there was a statistically significant correlation between scores obtained for HINT sentences in quiet and CNC words (r = 0.79) and BKB-SIN (r = –0.77), there was no *reliable relationship* between the measures that offered clinical or diagnostic utility. For example, considering the current SSA cut-off of 60 percent HINT sentences in quiet, individuals scoring within this range achieved scores between 8 and 53 percent for CNC words and between 9 and 21 dB SNR for BKB-SIN (Gifford et al., 2008). Thus, the committee is unable to accurately identify a conversion factor between HINT sentence recognition in quiet and other validated measures of speech recognition performance for at least two primary reasons: (1) there are no published datasets with large samples collected prospectively describing speech recognition scores across a number of measures, including HINT in quiet, and (2) the characteristics of the HINT sentences and the resultant non-normal, skewed distribution of scores in quiet limits the committee's ability to generate a reliable conversion value.

SUMMARY AND RECOMMENDATIONS

As described in Chapter 2, any measure of sentence recognition may be affected by talker rate, talker gender, enunciation, language complexity, a listener's native language, and various neurocognitive processes. Indeed, each measure of speech perception has its own set of strengths and weaknesses as it tests a diverse set of auditory, cognitive, and neurolinguistic abilities. It is for this reason that most professionals believe in the use of multiple measures of speech perception to fully capture the auditory and communication profile of the listener. The fields of audiology and otology have been moving toward the use of monosyllabic word recognition both for measuring cochlear implant candidacy and for tracking post-operative outcomes. In fact, a number of recent U.S. Food and Drug Administration (FDA)-approved clinical trials of new cochlear implant systems have used CNC monosyllabic word recognition as the primary measure for determining candidacy, with preoperative criteria ranging from 40 percent (Sladen et al., 2017; Wick et al., 2020; National Clinical Trial [NCT] 01337076; NCT 03236909) up to 60 percent correct (Roland et al., 2016; NCT 00678899; NCT 00747435). The use of monosyllabic words is already considered standard of care for speech audiometry in audiology clinics and is readily available. Additionally, within the context of determining candidacy for an intervention or for disability status, word recognition tasks will not penalize a listener for being able to "fill in the gaps" using higher level communication repair strategies. That is, word recognition tasks more accurately reflect the transmission of acoustic speech cues through the impaired auditory system.

The committee was tasked with recommending how scores from the identified tests can be compared with or converted to equivalent scores on the HINT. However, given the committee's concerns with the utility of the HINT and the limitations expressed in Chapter 3, such as ceiling effects and lack of availability, deriving equivalent scores on the HINT would produce scores with limited interpretation. Additionally, while it may be of value to have a common metric or a conversion equivalent in the presence of newer tests, the task is complicated by a lack of large research studies with head-to-head comparisons of the HINT with other tests. Methods developed in the context of psychologic testing, which can be generalized to any type of measurement, indicate the need for rigorous study designs to measure test scores on the same individuals in a single group (Dorans, 2007). It is also possible to link instruments that have not been administered to the same set of individuals, but the methods produce weaker data and require stronger assumptions. In summary, the lack of rigorous research studies prohibits completion of this task.

As noted in previous chapters, the current use of the HINT sentences as criteria for cochlear implantation may suffer from ceiling effects of the test materials, given modern technology and the lack of availability of test materials. Research may support an update of assessment of cochlear implementation via different materials. Speech assessment via sentences fundamentally differs from assessment via words because sentences offer context to the information, and context may result in improved scores in speech understanding. In Chapter 4 the committee made the following recommendation based on those factors and others, including the difficulty of obtaining the HINT, the shift in the cochlear implant community toward using word tests, and the fact that SSA already uses word tests for individuals with hearing loss who do not have a cochlear implant:

> Given the limitations of the Hearing in Noise Test, the committee recommends the use of a monosyllabic word recognition test to assess hearing loss in individuals treated with cochlear implantation, consistent with what the U.S. Social Security Administration currently uses to determine disability in adults and children with hearing loss not treated with cochlear implantation. Administration of the word test should include a full word list that is standardized and phonetically or phonemically balanced.

Examples of such tests, as of this writing, include the CNC words or the Northwestern University Test No. 6 for adults and the Phonetically Balanced Kindergarten or Lexical Neighborhood Test for children.

The Statement of Task also requests the committee "to identify and recommend generalized testing procedures and criteria for evaluating the level of functional hearing ability needed to make a disability determination in adults and children after cochlear implantation." Based on the information detailed in Chapters 2 through 5 and the committee's professional judgment:

> The committee recommends using the following presentation level and standardized test setup:
> - 60 dB SPL (sound pressure level) using hearing technology recommended for the individual that is functioning properly and adjusted to the individual's normal settings. In cases of single-sided deafness or asymmetric hearing loss, the non-implanted ear should not be occluded for testing,
> - The level should be calibrated for sound field presentation,
> - The test material should be recorded to ensure standardized administration,
> - Testing should occur in quiet in a sound-treated booth, and
> - The listener should be seated 1 meter from the loudspeaker at 0° azimuth.

Finally, the Statement of Task asks the committee

for the scores on hearing tests that correspond to a level of functional hearing ability that causes marked and severe functional limitation in a child or that prevents an adult from doing any gainful activity, regardless of his or her age, education, or work experience, and whether those scores can be expressed in a form comparable between hearing tests such as percentile or standard deviation from the norm.

The committee suggests that SSA use the same cut-off criteria for evaluating hearing loss in individuals with cochlear implants as the current Listing for hearing loss in individuals without cochlear implants. That cut-off aligns with the criteria used in the most recent FDA clinical trials for cochlear implants. Specifically, the FDA trials use a cut-off score of 40 percent correct or less in the ear to be implanted and 50 percent correct or less in the contralateral ear on a recorded monosyllabic word test presented at 60 dB sound pressure level, with A-weighting.

The committee recommends a score of 40 percent correct or less on a monosyllabic word test as the cut-off criterion for hearing loss in adults and children treated with cochlear implantation, consistent with the current U.S. Social Security Administration criterion for adults and children with hearing loss not treated with cochlear implantation.

The committee believes that should an individual with a cochlear implant continue to meet the criteria for cochlear implantation after they have been implanted with their device, they clearly have demonstrated that the cochlear implant has not provided significant benefit. As such, it is highly likely that the cochlear implant recipient has a disability related to hearing loss.

As mentioned, no single test can fully capture the broad neurological faculties that allow for speech and language understanding. Given that speech tests do not capture all of hearing function (see the section titled Considerations Beyond Auditory Testing in Chapter 4), the committee also notes that additional information from self-report or parent-report questionnaires may be useful for better characterizing an individual's real-world communicative functioning. Examples of such questionnaires, as of this writing, include the Cochlear Implant Quality of Life; the Cochlear Implant Function Index; the Nijmegen Cochlear Implant Questionnaire; the Hearing Handicap Inventory for Adults/Elderly; the Communication Profile for the Hearing Impaired; the Abbreviated Profile of Hearing Aid Benefit; the Speech, Spatial, and Qualities of Hearing Scale; the LittlEARS Auditory Questionnaire; the Meaningful Auditory Integration Scale (standard and the infant-toddler version); the Parents' Evaluation of Aural/Oral Performance of Children; and the Auditory Skills Checklist.

The recommendations of this committee were made based on the state of knowledge available to committee members at the time of writing. As advances in clinical practice, assessment measures, and hearing technology emerge, it is possible that a better measure for assessing significant disability will become available. Therefore, should more information become known in the future, it may be necessary to revisit the above recommendations.

REFERENCES

Carhart, R., and T. W. Tillman. 1970. Interaction of competing speech signals with hearing losses. *Archives of Otolaryngology* 91(3):273–279.

Carlson, M. L., N. S. Patel, N. M. Tombers, M. D. Dejong, A. I. Breneman, B. A. Neff, and C. L. W. Driscoll. 2017. Hearing preservation in pediatric cochlear implantation. *Otology and Neurotology* 38(6):e128–e133.

Cullington, H. E., and T. Aidi. 2017. Is the digit triplet test an effective and acceptable way to assess speech recognition in adults using cochlear implants in a home environment? *Cochlear Implants International* 18(2):97–105.

Dorans, N. J. 2007. Linking scores from multiple health outcome instruments. *Quality of Life Research* 16(Suppl 1):85–94.

Etymōtic Research. 2005. *BKB-SIN user's manual.* https://www.etymotic.com/downloads/dl/file/id/260/product/160/bkb_sintm_user_manual.pdf (accessed October 17, 2020).

Firszt, J. B., L. K. Holden, M. W. Skinner, E. A. Tobey, A. Peterson, W. Gaggl, C. L. Runge-Samuelson, and P. A. Wackym. 2004. Recognition of speech presented at soft to loud levels by adult cochlear implant recipients of three cochlear implant systems. *Ear and Hearing* 25(4):375–387.

Gifford, R. H., J. K. Shallop, and A. M. Peterson. 2008. Speech recognition materials and ceiling effects: Considerations for cochlear implant programs. *Audiology and Neurotology* 13(3):193–205.

Holder, J. T., L. M. Levin, and R. H. Gifford. 2018. Speech recognition in noise for adults with normal hearing: Age-normative performance for AzBio, BKB-SIN, and QuickSIN. *Otology & Neurotology* 39(10):e972–e978.

Killion, M. C., P. A. Niquette, G. I. Gudmundsen, L. J. Revit, and S. Banerjee. 2004. Development of a Quick Speech-in-Noise test for measuring signal-to-noise ratio loss in normal-hearing and hearing-impaired listeners. *Journal of the Acoustical Society of America* 116(4 I):2395–2405.

Litovsky, R., A. Parkinson, J. Arcaroli, and C. Sammeth. 2006. Simultaneous bilateral cochlear implantation in adults: A multicenter clinical study. *Ear and Hearing* 27(6):714–731.

Massa, S. T., and M. J. Ruckenstein. 2014. Comparing the performance plateau in adult cochlear implant patients using HINT and AzBio. *Otology & Neurotology* 35(4):598–604.

McArdle, R. A., R. H. Wilson, and C. A. Burks. 2005. Speech recognition in multitalker babble using digits, words, and sentences. *Journal of the American Academy of Audiology* 16(9):726–739.

Nilsson, M., S. D. Soli, and J. A. Sullivan. 1994. Development of the Hearing in Noise Test for the measurement of speech reception thresholds in quiet and in noise. *Journal of the Acoustical Society of America* 95(2):1085–1099.

Niquette, P., J. Arcaroli, L. Revit, A. Parkinson, S. Staller, M. Skinner, and M. Killion. 2003. *Development of the BKB-SIN test.* Paper presented at the Annual Meeting of the American Auditory Society, Scottsdale, AZ.

Roland, J. T., Jr., B. J. Gantz, S. B. Waltzman, and A. J. Parkinson. 2016. United States multicenter clinical trial of the cochlear nucleus hybrid implant system. *Laryngoscope* 126(1):175–181.

Sladen, D. P., R. H. Gifford, D. Haynes, D. Kelsall, A. Benson, K. Lewis, T. Zwolan, Q. J. Fu, B. Gantz, J. Gilden, B. Westerberg, C. Gustin, L. O'Neil, and C. L. Driscoll. 2017. Evaluation of a revised indication for determining adult cochlear implant candidacy. *Laryngoscope* 127(10):2368–2374.

Wick, C. C., M. J. Butler, L. H. Yeager, D. Kallogjeri, N. Durakovic, J. L. McJunkin, M. A. Shew, J. A. Herzog, and C. A. Buchman. 2020. Cochlear implant outcomes following vestibular schwannoma resection: Systematic review. *Otology & Neurotology* 41(9):1190–1197.

Wilson, R. H., R. A. McArdle, and S. L. Smith. 2007. An evaluation of the BKB-SIN, HINT, QuickSIN, and WIN materials on listeners with normal hearing and listeners with hearing loss. *Journal of Speech, Language, and Hearing Research* 50(4):844–856.